The Spirit of Budo
Old Traditions for Present-day Life

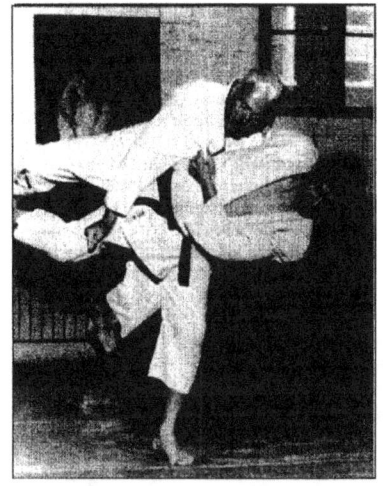

Trevor Leggett (left) with John Newman,
former Head of BBC Japanese Service

TREVOR LEGGETT ADHYATMA YOGA TRUST

Published in 2022 by Trevor Leggett Adhyatma Yoga Trust,
PO Box 362, King's Lynn, PE31 8WK, United Kingdom.
Website: www.tlayt.org

First published in English and Japanese in 1993 by Simul Press, Tokyo and in 1998 by Kegan Paul International, UK.

© Copyright Trevor Leggett Adhyatma Yoga Trust 1993, 1998, 2022.

All rights reserved. No part of this publication may be reproduced or utilised in any form or by any means, electronic or mechanical, including photocopying, recording, or by any information storage and retrieval systems, without the prior written permission of the publisher.

ISBN: 978-1-911467-17-5

CONTENTS

Foreward .... *v*
Preface .... *vii*

1 *Bujin* and the Gentleman 1
   The Spirit of Budo 3
   Sincerity 7
   Spectators 11
   Yin and Yang in Budo 15
   Inner Calm 21

2 Old Traditions Breathe Fire into Present-day Life 27
   Chivalry and Budo 29
   World Culture and Budo 33
   Impulsive Generosity 39
   On Humour 43
   Technical Training as a Means 47

3 Budo: Learning for Life 53
   Travel and Learn 55
   The Four Keys to Learning 61
   Dynamic Words 67
   Free from Fixed Ideas 71

4 **Dr. Jigoro Kano and Judo** 77
The Buddhist Ideal of Mutual Benefit 79
Bunbu Ryodo 文武両道 83
Judo in Real Life 87
The Will to Make It Happen 93

Notes 97
Glossary 99

Superscript numbers in the text (e.g.,[1], [2], etc.) refer to annotations provided in the Notes.
Brief descriptions on selected Judo terminology are given in the Glossary.

Foreword

The Trevor Leggett Adhyatma Yoga Trust ('TLAYT') is a registered charity established following the death of Trevor Leggett in August 2000. Its objectives are to promote the public knowledge of Yoga, Vedanta, Buddhism, Zen, Judo and shogi.

The trustees of TLAYT are delighted that The Spirit of Budo is available once again at an affordable price in both new softback and e-book editions. With the new edition of Kata Judo coming out shortly it means that all Trevor Leggett's books on Yoga, Zen, Judo and Shogi are now back in print again.

We hope that The Spirit of Budo, sub-titled 'Old Traditions for Present-day life', will be of interest and of value not only to practitioners of Judo and the other martial arts but also to all those interested in inner development and spiritual training generally.

The Trustees would like to thank Ben Anderson, a judo student and old friend of the author, for providing the Japanese calligraphy used on the front cover of this book.

The Trustees
Trevor Leggett Adhyatma Yoga Trust
April 2022

The Spirit of Budo

Preface

I began Judo in 1930 at the Budokwai in London, the oldest Judo club in Europe. I was 16 years old. Our teachers were the famous Yukio Tani, 4th dan, who was one of those who had introduced Judo to the West, and Gunji Koizumi, an art expert and also 4th dan. Tani came from a line of *jujutsu* teachers; his grandfather had given exhibitions before the shogun. While Tani never learnt English well, Koizumi was a cultured man who spoke and wrote good English.

The amazing success of *jujutsu* and Judo, demonstrated by Tani and others against Western wrestlers and boxers at the beginning of the century, had given them a magical reputation of wizardry in the physical realm. Phrases like 'Verily the soft controls the hard' *(ju yoku go o seisu)* became well known. Mitford's *Tales of Old Japan* and Kaiten Nukariya's[1] *Religion of the Samurai* led to idealization of the supposed 'living chivalry' of Japan. Even sceptical writers like H.G. Wells were impressed.

One evening I saw a pair of straw sandals in the Budokwai changing room. They belonged to Tani. I noticed that underneath each sole there was a small piece of metal fixed and wondered why it was there. Tani put the sandals on and walked a few steps with the metal making a tapping sound. He told me that the old samurai, like his grandfather, used to wear such sandals so that it would be impossible for them to steal silently up behind someone 'like a coward'. I was suitably impressed. He said, 'A true samurai washed his face with cold water only so that even after death it would remain firm'. For over 20 years afterwards, I washed and showered only in cold water, using hot water reluctantly for shaving.

I practised Judo hard and read about Japan—mostly idealistic stuff. I heard Dr. Jigoro Kano[2] speak when he came to London with Masami Takasaki and Sumiyuki Kotani. They confirmed my expectations, and I thought most Japanese must be like them. (I knew of course that Japanese bicycles and typewriters were of poor workmanship, though they were cheap. But by a sort of conjuring trick, this inconvenient fact disappeared down a mental trapdoor. Most idealists get adept at this trick.) So I wanted to be like the Japanese, more Japanese than the Japanese, if possible even *super-Japanese*.

Then I got a big surprise from a young Japanese businessman. He was marvellously skilful at Judo and gave me lessons in advanced technique. In turn, I gave him lessons in golf and took him to some good courses. One day I told him never to stand closer than about ten yards when another player is making a fairway shot. 'That's golf etiquette', I said.

Afterwards he thanked me effusively, adding: 'As we are friends, I want to ask a favour. Please tell me, without any hesitation, about any points of behaviour where I make a mistake. I shall not think it rude; I shall be grateful. I want to behave like a perfect English gentleman'.

I could hardly believe my ears. I was trying to be like a Japanese, while he was trying to be like an Englishman, or rather like our imagined paragons of Japanese and Englishman. Still, as a matter of fact, we both worked very hard to actualize at least some part of these ideals. Moreover, we had learnt something from each other: there was also great value in our own native traditional culture, on which we (like many young men in all generations) had previously turned our backs.

After World War II, in which he had fought on the mainland and I in Southeast Asia, we met occasionally. We used to grin at each other at the thought of our previous naiveté. We now knew the dark sides of our former ideals as well as the bright and dark sides of our own culture. Yet on the deepest level, something remained. He became a successful politician, though contemptuous of what he called the 'small-minded corruption' he found in the world of politics. He told me once that a few of them were trying to change it to something like the British model. 'But it will take a long time; everything is interlinked'.

Preface

In 1946 I had the chance to become head of the Japanese Service of the BBC. We were broadcasting to young people in Japan, like that young businessman friend of years before, but we did not broadcast just good points about Britain. I did not want to create illusions. After all, if we know someone who talks only of his good points, never mentioning his failures, we do not like him, do we? So we broadcast about our difficulties and struggles as well. Our frankness appealed to listeners. The Japanese Service was very successful, and many of our scripts were later published as books by the Simul Press in the Lion Series and by other publishers. This achievement was unique to the Japanese Service.

Broadcasting to Japan was my professional life. I took part once a week, answering letters from our listeners. I remained as head of the Japanese Service for nearly 25 years, refusing promotion to higher administrative posts. But I wanted to do something in the reverse direction. I believed that Judo was a good introduction to Japanese tradition, and with the prestige of my 6th dan from the Kodokan I taught most of the British Judo teachers. Many of them learnt Japanese, spoken and written, went to Japan and wrote books afterwards about Japan.

As Judo became an international sport, I grew disappointed and predicted that the ideals of Dr. Kano would be largely lost. And they have been largely lost. The concession of making a standing bow, instead of the traditional *zarei* (a sitting bow) symbolized this loss. It was a misunderstanding of the psychology of foreigners, most of whom would have liked to preserve the old traditions, as they have been preserved to some extent in fencing. Judo as a mere sport has lost its main original purpose set out by Dr. Kano—training for life. Dr. Kano, Takasaki and Kotani never showed outwardly that they were experts in Judo, though a trained eye could see it. We were impressed by their calm demeanour, and British Judo men of my generation never swaggered. Nowadays some have begun to swagger as in Japan. They may be first-rate at technique on the tatami but are only second-rate at Judo.

Judo practice can be no more than an introduction to the much deeper Budo spirit. Some outside observers (and even some Japanese) deny that it exists. When Japan was in ruins just after World War II, there was a view that its future lay in becoming a tourist lotus land. Its wonderful decorative charm would make it a holiday centre for the world. *Yamato-damashii* (the Japanese spirit), it was said, had originally meant the ability to appreciate cherry blossoms, and so it would be again. Budo would vanish. I never believed this. I felt that Budo would not vanish but would show itself in new forms. (Perhaps the present excellence of Japanese products is one such form.)

In 1947 I went round the secondhand bookshops in the Kanda district of Tokyo, which had miraculously survived the bombs, and bought many books on Budo and Zen. These books were now almost given away, and the whole group of ideals had been discredited. I began to translate some of these materials—no easy task. Already in 1946 I had published some short essays in small magazines. At first, editors asked for articles about the decorative arts or about 'how Japan has changed'. But quite soon they were attracted to the theme of Budo. One of my earlier writings, 'The Maxims of Saigo[3]', became rather well known. In 1956 my *First Zen Reader*, a collection of translations, was brought out by Charles Tuttle in Tokyo and had a big success. It was followed by a number of other writings—translations and some essays of my own.

This book consists of 18 articles which have appeared in the monthly *Budo* magazine and are reproduced here by the kind permission of the editor and my friend Mr. Kisaburo Watanabe. My thanks go to Mr. Katsuo Tamura, President of the Simul Press, for his co-operation.

It may seem daring for a foreigner to write on Budo. Yet there are parallels in history. Ask anyone for the composer who uniquely represents the spirit of Hungary, and they will answer 'Franz Liszt'. But he was taken from Hungary when a baby and could hardly speak a word of Hungarian: he was in fact a foreigner. Still, even true Hungarians find his *Hungarian Rhapsodies* worth listening to. May it be so with the 18 essays which are presented in this book.

Trevor P. Leggett

November 1993

1
Bujin and the Gentleman

The Spirit of Budo

The Spirit of Budo

In this first essay I would like to recall how an Englishman, who was brought up 70 years ago in the traditional way, viewed the Budo spirit in Japan in about 1940, and to tell you how he sees the Budo spirit today.

First of all, I should say a few words about the persistence of the ideas. When I was young, there were ideas of being a gentleman; doing one's duty honourably and keeping calm under all circumstances were the main things in life. Culture was less important. In the romantic novels read by young people then, the plot often centred round some conflict of duty: the hero's problem was just to discover what his duty was. Then he would do it and marry the heroine. She would never marry anyone who did not carry out his duty.

In my teens, I did not much like these traditional ideas. They seemed to me rather narrow and boring. I was interested in Communism for a short time; it had some ideas that seemed good. But then I perceived that though there were genuine idealists among the lower ranks of Communists, the ones at the top were simply using the ideas as a means to personal power. In Britain at least, they mostly hated each other. This was confirmed when Stalin began killing most of his early associates.

Taking a New Look at Budo

In search of adventure at age 21, I managed to spend a year abroad, mostly in Germany and Czechoslovakia. I made my own living and did not take any money from my parents. To my surprise, I found that the Continental people expected me, as an Englishman, to behave in the traditional way.

They expected me to be calm, very polite, and a good sportsman. If I said or did something 'out of character', they were disappointed. I began to feel that I was like an actor cast in a certain role which was not my real nature. On my side, I discovered many things. For instance, I was surprised to see the reverence of the Germans for learning: in Britain then, learned men were respected, but not reverenced as they were in Germany.

But I was now meeting people who were not calm, not fair, not patient, and who did not feel personally responsible for their actions. As long as they followed orders, they did not feel responsible. As I got wider experience of the world, gradually I came to see that the traditional British ideas of calm, fairness, patience and responsibility were more important than I had thought.

In the same way, when I went to Japan in 1938 at the age of 24, I found that many young Japanese did not like their traditions of Budo, which were then strongly encouraged.

And in 1950, when I visited the secondhand bookshops in Kanda, they were full of discarded old books on Budo, which seemed to be completely discredited. I bought a number of them. I believed, however, that the valuable points of Budo would revive and come to be recognized by Japanese as part of their identity. To some extent, this has happened.

After my first return to Japan I went back every two or three years up to 1964, when I had a year in Japan. Very soon after my first post-war visit, I noticed that though there was conscious adoption of many Western things, especially American, on the films and radio—and then on TV—there began to appear *chambara* dramas featuring sword fights. Although the background notions of such films were dismissed as feudal to be rejected by a modern nation, they still appeared in these media, becoming more and more numerous.

They were classed as mere entertainment, and so of course they were. But I asked myself: 'Why is this kind of entertainment so popular?' Some Japanese friends of mine who were Communist in outlook still used to watch them. I felt that the people were seeking their own identity, and I guessed that they would ultimately find it in aspects of their own history.

Many Japanese were amazed to find that foreigners admired Japanese traditional culture. Slowly, over the next 20 or 30 years, the Japanese came to know the defects in the foreign cultures they admired, and they slowly turned again to look at their own.

One of the things they looked at was the spirit of Budo.

They could see that Judo had lost something important in its spirit as it became an international sport. It was no longer a training for life as Dr. Jigoro Kano had intended as the founder. It had tended to become a competitive sport mainly practised in order to do well in competitions. Western coaches took it up enthusiastically, applying the training methods used in athletics and competitive sports. Western coaches simply laughed at things like the Judo *kangeiko,* or midwinter training: it might be good for training soldiers, but it had no meaning in sports. To get the best results was the aim of sports; *kangeiko* would not help to get good results.

Inner Calm and Resolution

For over 10 years from 1952 at the 100-tatami London Budokwai, I ran a weekend class for black belts, who came from all over Britain every week to attend. There were about 60 of them, and they became the Judo teachers of the next generation. We held a *kangeiko* every year. An athletics coach once asked me, 'What benefit do they get from this?'

'It is a training in being able to face difficult circumstances', I told him, 'with inner calm and resolution'.

'Well, what is the good of that?' he asked. 'The Judo competitions will be held, like all athletic competitions, in reasonable circumstances—not in the very early morning in midwinter with the windows open'.

'Yes, but in your athletic competitions, have you ever noticed how very nervous many of the competitors are?' I asked. 'The smallest thing seems to upset them and put them off'. And I gave some examples of tennis stars who lost their temper on the court and screamed and shouted because of some imagined fault of the umpire.

He admitted this but said, 'They still win'.

'They may win at tennis, but they do not win at life', I replied. 'Their tennis does not help them in life; it does not give them a calm inner will. That is more important than their technique. This is a central point in our

Judo training. We do study technique, but we study inner training which is more important. This spirit runs through the Japanese tradition in all the Knightly Ways, which are called Budo'.

He got excited and cried: 'Give me one example where the inner training shows itself more effectively than a superior technique. I challenge you to give me just one example!'

So I told him a story I had heard in Kyoto.

> Japanese archers draw to the shoulder. When the bow is fully stretched, the right hand is level with the right shoulder. Western archers draw to the cheek or to the ear. The Japanese draw is fuller and thus more powerful than the classical Western one, but it is in general less accurate. An expert American archer, who visited Japan in the 1930s, showed a Japanese master that his Western style was more accurate than the Japanese. They went together to the range, and the American could get slightly better results on the target.
>
> The American offered to give him some lessons, but to his surprise the unimpressed Japanese master said: 'You may do a bit better on the range, but that is not the point'. The American was understandably annoyed and retorted: 'Then what is the point of archery, if it is not to get the best results?'
>
> 'Well, let us take up our bows and three arrows and go to opposite ends of the range', said the Japanese master. 'Then let us shoot at each other. If you are the better archer, you will win'. The challenge was declined. 'That is the point of our archery', he added. The Western archer left in silence.

So did the athletics coach, after he had listened to this. He told me later that it had given him a new perspective on what he was teaching.

Sincerity

In 1938, my first year in Japan, I noticed how often the word 'sincerity' came up. Sometimes I was surprised at how it was used. For instance, before leaving Britain I had met the Japanese ambassador in London, Mr. Mamoru Shigemitsu. He walked with a stick, and I assumed that he had probably been in a car accident. Later on, I was told that he had had a bomb thrown at him by a Japanese nationalist. Many years later, I heard that Mr. Shigemitsu had met this bomb thrower, after he had finished his dozen years in prison.

The Japanese press asked Mr. Shigemitsu how he felt about this man, and he replied something like this: 'I have no resentment against him, because I feel that he was sincere in his beliefs'. A British politician would not say this. In fact, after an attempt was made to kill her by a bomb, Mrs. Margaret Thatcher said: 'These people may be sincere in their beliefs, but those beliefs are completely wrong. They are half-mad, and they are cowardly murderers'.

We can say that most British people would feel like this. So I felt it strange that some Japanese were more impressed by the sincerity of a person than by his words. If a person was very earnest, they respected him.

Being Sincere vs. Being Right

After Judo practice I regularly went out with some Japanese student friends. They wanted to practise their English, and I wanted to practise my Japanese. So the conversation was a mixture of broken English and broken Japanese. Occasionally we were joined by others, who wanted to meet a foreigner. (There were not many of us in Japan in those days.)

On one occasion, one of these Japanese students began a long talk about the world: 'The old name for Japan was *sumera-no-kuni,* and world civilization began in Sumer in Mesopotamia. Sumer was obviously a mistake for *sumera,* and therefore world civilization began in Japan'. He said all this very earnestly, not aggressively, but often looking at me, evidently hoping to convince me. I could follow enough of his Japanese and English to understand him. He repeated himself often, which made it easier.

It was obvious nonsense, and I expected someone to say so or at least interrupt him. But they listened to it all with respect.

After he had gone, I asked one of them, 'Surely you don't believe that sort of thing, do you?' 'No, I don't', he replied. 'But we feel that he is very sincere. We generally respect a sincere man, even if he is talking nonsense'.

Later I asked a Japanese professor whom I was helping with an English translation. He looked a little embarrassed and said: 'These ideas are dreamed up by some ideologues; they publish them in little magazines, and that man had probably read an article about it. In our present wartime climate, it can be dangerous to laugh at such ideas. Apart from that, we Japanese are impressed by someone very sincere, because we feel he must have put in a good deal of his life into his belief. So some of us think that he must know quite a lot about it, and probably he is right on at least one or two points'.

Ever since then I have noticed this Japanese attitude again and again, and I still do today. There is a big contrast with the British standpoint. Not so many British people think like that. We feel that someone who concentrates on a single subject may often become too narrow. He may know that particular subject, but he forgets everything else. Although the one-pointed action is very impressive, it sometimes happens that the outer situation has changed. Then the action has become meaningless.

But the Japanese born in Meiji believed that sincerity has a value in itself, and that it is a sort of guarantee that an action is somehow right. Many young Japanese feel opposed to the old attitudes, but unconsciously they are strongly influenced by them.

Virtues of Sincerity

An Indian scholar whom I knew very well once told me a story about a typical Japanese born in Meiji. This Indian lived in Japan in the early part of this century and lectured on Indian philosophy at a few universities in Tokyo. He was a great friend of Prof. Junjiro Takakusu[4].

When the late Emperor Hirohito was crown prince, it was arranged that he would have an hour's lecture on each of the world's great religions from some outstanding authority. Prof. Takakusu was asked to select the lecturer for Hinduism, and he chose this Indian professor. (He told me that the young Crown Prince had listened for an hour without moving, and that at the end he asked intelligent questions.)

This Indian scholar believed that India should not seek independence from Britain too soon. He said that Britain could do much to organize India, and that India would give spiritual truth to Britain and, through Britain, to the West. In previous centuries India had given Mahayana Buddhism to China and, through China, to Japan. Mahayana Buddhism had been the greatest civilizing force the world had ever known. Something similar could happen in this century, but in a Western direction.

He openly expressed these views, and this brought him into conflict with men like Mitsuru Toyama, who wanted to help a revolution in India. He twice met Toyama who respected his courage and sincerity. He also got to know one of the Japanese, who led the so-called Free India movement in Japan. One day he asked this Japanese how he had become interested in a movement for India. The man then told a story which I could believe only because he was a Japanese. If he had been a man of any other nation, I could never have accepted it. This man said:

> I was walking through Tokyo one afternoon with nothing particular to do. I passed a small hall, which had a badly written notice advertising a lecture by some foreigner. No title was given, but I went in out of curiosity. I was the only one in the hall. A Japanese came in with an Indian and said that unfortunately the interpreter had not come; so the lecture would be given in English. Then he left. The Indian got up and addressed the single

listener with as much passion and force as if he had been speaking to a full hall. I did not understand a word. Afterwards he came up and spoke to me, but I could only spread my hands.

I left him waiting for his guide to come back. But I was so impressed by his sincerity that I determined first to find out what he had been talking about and then to devote my life to it. I have done so.

The Indian scholar who told me this story said that this Japanese man was, as he put it, 'a member of a group whose programme was world domination by assassination. He was no ordinary man'.

The British respect sincerity too, but we feel it is often wasted. Unless it brings something good, it is wasted. Unless people know about it, it is wasted. However, Japanese often feel that sincerity is a value in itself, whether it is known about or not. Often a poem will express an attitude perfectly. So I will quote two poems, one English and one Japanese, to bring out the difference in our attitude to sincerity. The first is from the famous *Elegy Written in a Country Churchyard* by Thomas Gray (1716-1771):

> Full many a gem of purest ray serene,
> The dark unfathom'd caves of ocean bear:
> Full many a flower is born to blush unseen,
> And waste its sweetness on the desert air.

The second is by a Japanese poet whose name I do not know:

> Not for the sake of a beholder,
> In the deep mountains the cherry blooms
> Out of the sincerity of its heart.

Spectators

Traditionally in Britain there have been two sorts of games: cricket, golf and fencing, which were associated with gentlemen, and soccer and wrestling, which were associated with the masses.

In the so-called gentlemanly games, there was very little applause. At a cricket match 50 years ago, there would be only some occasional discreet clapping when a batsman scored a fine stroke. As the game became internationalized, there were audiences in foreign countries who did not have this tradition of self-control, and the behaviour of the onlookers became wilder. To this day, fencing is strict in its control of audience behaviour: anyone who attempted to barrack would be ejected. In golf, the foreign professionals comment on the good behaviour of British onlookers. They do not crowd the players, as they do in some tournaments abroad.

In 1939 I watched and took part in contests at the Kodokan and elsewhere; there was no cheering or clapping from the spectators. (It must also be said that the conduct of the contestants is often a good deal rougher today.) Judo was still regarded as no mere sport but a character training; the whole atmosphere was correspondingly serious and dignified. All foreigners who saw it were most impressed. I find it disappointing and regrettable to see how today the attitude has changed into a sporting event. It is not even a dignified and self-controlled sporting event, because the ideal of the sportsman itself has also degenerated.

I believe that if Japan readopted its own traditional standards of behaviour at contests within Japan itself, it would have an effect on the world attitudes to Judo.

Shogi and Western Chess

Where Japan has kept to its traditions, the world has in fact been impressed. For instance, there are few games where there is less action than *shogi, go* or Western chess. The *shogi* championships are fought out in a quiet room with a referee and recorders. At most three or four honoured guests are allowed to watch. I have been one of them; it was an honour. I was invited because I had just received a 5th dan at *shogi* from the Japan Shogi Federation. The then champion Yasuharu Oyama wrote the certificate in his own hand, and I keep it as a rare treasure.

In Japan, *shogi* is much more popular than chess is in Europe and America, though in the former Soviet Union it is encouraged. Our newspapers do not have a daily chess column, while the Japanese papers have a daily *shogi* and *go* column. Yet though *shogi* is so popular, the Japanese recognize that the players ought to have quiet and privacy for their tournament games. Those of the general public who want to watch the moves of the games sit in a separate hall, where the changing position is shown, move by move, on a very big display board. A *shogi* master comments on the moves to explain the strategy to the audience. There is excitement in the public hall, but the players in their silent room are protected from any disturbance.

Contrast this with the Western world chess championships, which take place in some enormous hall, in front of hundreds of people. Though they are spectators, they cannot see the position on the actual board, which is of course only the size of a small tabletop. The moves are shown on a huge display board at the end of the hall. They can also see the players, but it is quite meaningless.

The players are distracted by cameras and camera lights. Sometimes the spectators clap and even cheer, if they think a good move has been made. It is not so much a test of chess as a test of the calm of the players. Bobby Fischer, an American and perhaps the greatest genius of chess, won the world championship, but then gave up championship chess because of the constant disturbances during matches. The Western chess championship arrangements are an example of great stupidity and vulgarity. The audiences simply look at the two players from a distance.

In 1978 a Russian player named Korchnoi, who was out of favour with the Soviet authorities, played the champion Viktor Karpov, who was liked by them. Korchnoi complained that a mysterious Russian spectator, sitting in the sixth row of seats, was looking at him fixedly, trying to hypnotize him. The press investigated and found that the man was Dr. Zoukhar, a Russian government psychiatrist, who could not play chess. He was simply sitting there, staring, and Korchnoi (a very irritable nervous man) said that it upset him. Under the rules, the referee could not interfere: Dr. Zoukhar was simply sitting there quietly. But finally he was persuaded to sit further back. He or his Soviet government employers realized that though he was successful in upsetting Korchnoi, the publicity was becoming unfavourable.

If we compare these amazing happenings with the atmosphere of Japanese *go* and *shogi*, we get a very high estimate of the civilized and gentlemanly Japanese arrangements. I have described the example of chess, because it shows how a purely intellectual game, with no action at all, can be taken over by the desire for a public display which can be a focus for group rivalry. The game is no longer for its own sake; it is simply a means to show a superiority of one group over another.

True Sportsmanship

The true spirit of sportsmanship is appreciation of the game itself. The game must not be a means of national or group superiority. In the English soccer, the teams were generally representative of a particular town. Soccer originally did not have a strong tradition of sportsmanship; it was the sport of the masses. So the crowd of spectators was divided into two parties; each would applaud a goal by their own side but would be silent when the other side scored.

But in a cricket match, the spectators—though supporting one side—would applaud a skilful stroke by one of the opposing batsmen. The true sportsman could appreciate an opponent's skill as well as his own. He could rise above mere partisanship and view the game from above, as it were. This ability to rise above the immediate situation was one of the most valuable assets given by sport. Of course, the sportsman tries to win and tries very hard. But he is independent of winning or losing. He is not overly elated when he wins; he is not depressed when he loses. This attitude, if it is cultivated, gives him a calm independence even in the most dangerous situations in life.

We can say that this sporting attitude came to be appreciated in amateur soccer also, but not by the spectators at professional matches. There the sport has become an entertainment, mixed up with a sort of tribal hatred of the supporters of the other teams. The same has come to be true of some other sports: in the Olympics it is clear that for many of the teams the only thing that matters is victory— getting medals for their own country.

As cricket has become international, the behaviour of spectators shows that they do not understand the purpose of sport at all. They want their side to win; if disappointed, they invade the pitch and even attack the players. It must be said that the behaviour of Japanese spectators is in general much better than that of the Western 'football hooligans', among whom the British are some of the worst.

But, as a matter of fact, the whole business of making sport into an entertainment is a big loss. It becomes like horse racing. The spectators at a horse race do not themselves run; they just watch and bet. In 'entertainment sport', the spectators may never have played the game at all. They identify themselves with the players, but they do not themselves play. They get nothing out of it as a training for life.

The 'entertainment players' or 'national representative players' also get nothing out of the sport. They have no idea of self-control; they cannot rise above elation if they win, or depression if they lose. A good tennis player, even a champion, is just a tennis player; he may be no good at life at all. Today, his sport gives him no inner training except concentration and skill with a racket.

Against this, a good sportsman, though his technical skill may be not high, learns an inner balance that enables him to face the changes of life without inner disturbance. He does not get confused in a crisis: he can meet unexpected bad luck, or good luck, with the same calm smile and cool judgement. This is the true meaning of sport, not breaking world records in front of a passive audience who never takes part in sport themselves.

Yin and Yang in Budo

In some texts of traditional schools of Budo like the *Itto-ryu*[5], there is a distinction between the Budo of yin and the Budo of yang. I first heard about this from a Judo teacher, long before I could read the Budo texts. It confirmed an impression that had been growing in me that there are two kinds of Budo. This is the sort of thing that some of the traditions taught:

> Before a combat, the swordsman of yin is perfectly calm. His expression does not change; he does not defy the enemy. He does not stare at the opponent wide-eyed or try to intimidate him with feints. He does not come forward with little steps, as if crossing a single-plank bridge, but he walks as if on a wide road, with a perfectly normal posture. This is a master who can hardly be defeated.
>
> The swordsman of yang, on the other hand, has an expression which would seem to crush rocks, has an aggressive posture, stares wide-eyed and tries to intimidate the opponent by feints and glaring at him. He advances and retreats awkwardly; his heart is agitated and he is weak.

One of the texts added, I remember, that the yin fighter can, if necessary, imitate the fury of the yang. But inwardly he remains calm.

From my first introduction to the ideas of Budo, I have been mentally dividing the practice, pictures, texts and traditions into two kinds of Budo. I used to think of them as Narrow Budo and Wide Budo.

Calm Prevails Over Fury

In making a Judo throw in contest, the Narrow school used to give this advice:

'Have only one idea—to cast yourself completely into the throw. Have no doubts about whether it will succeed or not. Simply give a loud shout and throw your whole body into it. If you allow yourself to have even the smallest doubt about the throw, or even a thought about anything else, your movement will become hesitant. You have to be one-pointed, completely one-pointed. The throw must be the whole world, and you feel you are throwing the whole world'.

I saw this demonstrated by Judo men of 4th and 5th dan, and I practised with some of them. The first months of this sort of practice at the Kodokan and other *dojo* training halls in 1939 gave me experience of how effective the Narrow Budo can be. I mentally associate it with the picture of scowling samurai giving a loud yell as he rushes forward. I saw it—and still see it today—in innumerable *chambara* (sword fights) films and strip cartoons.

The same sort of thing appeared in fields outside Budo. I saw and heard orators who just shouted the same thing again and again with total conviction. It was something which they believed with their whole heart. They would not permit any analysis or discussion of it. In an argument, they repeated their point of view with increasing noise each time. Their attitude would become threatening and could often overcome opposition by shouting.

But I was interested in the comment in the Budo texts about the yang fighter: 'his heart is agitated and he is weak'. At first, this seemed untrue. So often the furious fighter does overawe the opponent and wins. But I noticed cases where the opponent is not overawed by the ferocious expression and furious attack of a yang fighter. In those cases, the calm man could often win decisively.

I learnt from my elder brother that there is something like this in boxing, though of course they do not have words like yin and yang. He was an expert amateur boxer. He was so good when he was young that he even had an offer from a boxing promoter, who promised him a good career in boxing. In fact, he became a successful aircraft engineer. In his youth the job took him to some rough areas of London, and occasionally he got into fights.

A few times, he told me, it had been quite dangerous; a local bully did not like the young chap from London. Once my brother did get quite badly injured. He remarked to me that a boxer does not have much real advantage outside the ring, among tables and chairs, without boxing gloves. He said:

'Your Judo would be much better, I suppose. In a real fight, I can't do much if he manages to get into a clinch. I have to knock the spirit out of him with one punch at the very beginning. But if I hit him on the jaw, that may damage my hand too. And it's not easy to knock him out with a solar plexus punch, unless he's got his hands up. An experienced fighter does not come forward with hands high. And perhaps he recognizes a boxer; something about my stance probably. So he does not try to hit at all; he tries to get close and smother my arms by holding. That's his strategy.

'But I've got my own strategy, which always works. As he comes forward cautiously, I spit in his face. Then he goes mad and runs at me with his fists up to smash my face—it's a basic instinct. And he runs right on to my fist'.

When I heard this, I thought of the yin and yang. My brother's method—not very refined, I admit—turned a cool calculating opponent into a furious demon. The opponent's surface yin was turned into yang, with a disastrous result for him.

British people have our yang fighters—the football hooligans, for instance—but in general it is the yin fighter who is admired.

Admiral Drake and Tadamasa

We have a famous story about Admiral Drake, the British naval hero who lived at the end of the 16th century. The Spanish king equipped and sent a great fleet, called the Armada, to attack Britain. He had good reasons to expect the attack but did not know when the Spanish fleet would come. It must have been like Hojo Tokimune[6] waiting for the Mongol fleet. Drake was playing a game of bowls when a messenger rushed in with the news: 'A great fleet had been sighted!'

'We have time to finish the game', Drake said calmly. And they finished the game. He then joined the British fleet, which then defeated the Spanish. (We were helped, just as the Japanese had been, by the weather.)

This story is probably not true. I admit that when I heard it as a small boy, I thought Drake was a bit of a fool. He ought to have gone straight to take command of the British fleet. But the purpose of the story was to give an example of absolute self-control and confidence.

A better example, which I sometimes use when lecturing on Japan, is the way the tea ceremony was performed even just before a battle. British people are always very surprised to hear about it; they find it almost unbelievable. The tea ceremony requires very delicate precision of movement. For instance, unless it is set down with absolute precision, the delicate little tea ladle will fall over. The slightest shaking of the hand or other signs of nervousness will be clearly seen. 'So they do it as a demonstration of perfect calm—inner and outer'. When I say these words, some of the Western audience give a little gasp of surprise and admiration.

Japanese who intend to go abroad should learn a few things like this about the Budo of yin. They should find a translation and memorize a few sentences so that they can explain it without difficulty in the foreign language. It will be very interesting to the foreigners whom they meet.

There is an account of an early tea ceremony not well known even to historians of Budo. *Shonan katto-roku*[7] of the Muromachi era—which I translated into English and published in Britain in 1985—gives a brief description of a warrior of yin and a Zen follower, who imitated a warrior of yang:

> Tadamasa, a senior retainer of Hojo Takatoki, the regent, had the Buddhist name Anzan (quiet mountain). He was a keen Zen follower and for 23 years came and went to the meditation hall for laymen at the Kenchoji temple. When the fighting broke out everywhere in 1331, he was wounded in one engagement, but in spite of the pain galloped to Kenchoji to see Suzan, the 27th teacher there. A tea ceremony was going on at the temple, and the teacher seeing the man in armour come in quickly put a teacup in front of him and asked, 'How is this?'

The warrior at once crushed it under his foot and said, 'Heaven and earth are broken up altogether'.

'When heaven and earth are broken up, how is it with you?' asked the teacher. Anzan stood with his hands crossed over his breast. The teacher hit him, and he involuntarily cried out from the pain of his wounds.

'Heaven and earth not quite broken up yet', the teacher said.

The drum sounded from the camp across the mountain, and Tadamasa galloped quickly back. The next evening he came again, covered with blood, to see the teacher. He came out and asked again, 'When heaven and earth are broken up, how is it with you?'

Supporting himself on his blood-stained sword, Anzan gave a great *katsu* (loud yell) and died standing in front of the teacher.

The Spirit of Budo

Inner Calm

When I am asked how to tell the difference between Japanese and Chinese, I sometimes answer:

'In general, Japanese are more self-controlled. They talk less excitedly, speak in lower tone, move their bodies less and do not use many gestures. They usually do not interrupt each other. They seem a rather placid people'.

'But remember', I add, 'this applies to the exterior'. 'Within, the Japanese may be irritable, nervous, quarrelsome and deeply emotional. It is only that at ordinary times they do not like to show it. Only at exceptional times, when they are really roused, they do show it'.

I sometimes explain that the ordinary word for 'Excuse me' in Japanese is *shitsurei*. *Rei* means something like a ceremony, orderly and harmonious; *shitsu* means losing it or breaking it. So the word *shitsurei* means: 'I am doing something out of order, breaking the smooth surface conduct which is so important in Japan'.

Of course, such generalizations are made about all nations. It is a curious fact that though there is truth in them, they never seem to apply to the individuals whom the foreigner meets. For instance, before I went to live in Germany in 1935, I had read that Germans speak more loudly than most other nations. So I was prepared to meet verbally booming Germans. But in fact, most of the Germans whom I met in Frankfurt used to speak to me rather quietly. So I thought, 'Oh, the book was wrong'. I had lived there a little time and noticed that when the Germans spoke to each other, they used a louder voice. At first I thought they were always angry with each other. Then I realized that this was their normal voice. When they spoke to me, they spoke gently and slowly, using simple German so that I could understand easily. I was a special case. The book had been right.

Similarly, we can read that French people are quick to understand. When you talk to a Frenchman, often he will grasp the point of what you are saying, before you have finished your sentence. French people (like Indians) love argument and debate. So he does not want to agree with what you are saying. And before you have finished your sentence, he has understood your meaning and disagrees. He interrupts: 'Mais non, mais non!' (But no, but no!) British and Japanese feel that this is rather rude, but other French people do not mind it at all. They enjoy it. Television watching is not so popular in France as in most countries. It is said that this is because one cannot interrupt the television by saying, 'Mais non, mais non!'

The English too are seen by others as rather strange. A Spaniard once said to me:

'Your English way of talking is like your English weather—dull with not much sunshine. You use exactly the same voice to talk about a football match as about a terrible earthquake or fire; it's as though the earthquake or fire is no more important than a football match. Or perhaps a football match is as important to you as an earthquake or fire. You English talking together are like a full orchestra in which only the violas play!'

Similarly, to an Indian, the Japanese way of talking seems rather inexpressive, especially in Kyoto. On the surface at least, it is calm. A British poet, visiting Japan, remarked that the speech of Japanese women with children made him think of the song of small birds: it was so musical.

Calm but Resolute

The outer calm, which so impresses visitors to Japan, is part of an external gloss, which may be no deeper than a thin layer. When we live in Japan with Japanese people, we discover how paper-thin it often is. Then some foreigners become disillusioned. In their first few weeks, they see only the outside—the ceremonial order and the happy *matsuri* (festival). Later, after having lived some time in Japan, they find out what happens after the *matsuri* is over. It can be something quite different: confusion and turmoil, bitter hatreds and infighting and even worse.

But suppose they stay still longer and are able to go much deeper into the Japanese spirit. Usually they can only do this through real skill in one of the traditional Japanese arts. (In the same way, foreigners can make real English friends by becoming skilful at a traditional English sport like golf. But they must be really good.) Through Budo especially, a foreigner can come into touch with a very deep calm, much deeper than the superficial dignity of ceremonies or social politeness. When we first find out about this level, it is a great surprise to us.

When I was in Japan in 1939, I was introduced to an old man who, when he was young, had been a friend of another old man, who when young had been a friend of Saigo Takamori. The old Japanese told me that even at the height of fame, Saigo lived a very simple life. Sometimes someone would come and ask to sit with Saigo. The man would be admitted to the room where Saigo was. But neither Saigo nor the visitor would say a word. After about 15 minutes, the visitor would bow deeply and go, still without a word being spoken. 'It is known that if we come here and sit with Great Saigo for a few minutes, all the difficulties and indecisions in our heart will be solved', he added. 'We come here feeling anxious, and we go away calm and resolute'.

When I heard this, I found it almost incredible. I could not think of any similar case in Western history, except for a few saints. And even they generally said a word or two: blessings or something like that. The idea of just coming, sitting in silence and then going seems very strange to us. Of course, to most Japanese today, it would be a strange behaviour, but most of them have a vague understanding of it.

Saigo: A Man of Spiritual Strength

I was interested in the story and tried to read about Saigo. I asked my teacher of Japanese at the British embassy if he could find some short pieces about Saigo. He found a couple of books and selected a few fairly easy passages. I could improve my Japanese by studying them in advance and then with him. This was much more interesting than extracts from newspapers, which some other language students used.

I remember reading about three samurai who had approached Katsu Kaishu[8], asking for a letter of introduction to Saigo in Kyushu. Katsu suspected that these samurai intended to kill Saigo but wrote a note introducing them, in which he warned Saigo of what he suspected. He sealed it and gave it to their leader. Assuming that it was a mere introduction, they went to Kyushu, to Saigo's small house. When he came out in his simple clothes, they assumed that he was a servant. They handed him the letter, saying: 'Give this to your master'.

To their surprise, he opened it, read it and said: 'So you've come to kill me? All the way from the capital—quite a journey'. And he laughed. They looked at each other in bewilderment and then left.

'But why didn't they kill him?' I asked my teacher. He was an intellectual man and looked a bit embarrassed. I think he was afraid that I would find it incredible. Finally he said awkwardly: 'Well, it is difficult to explain, but some of those Meiji heroes had a sort of... a sort of what we call spiritual strength'.

I felt I had met something deep in the Japanese character. Later I read something about the attack on Admiral Kantaro Suzuki in the February 26, 1936 attempt at a coup. The assassin, Captain Teruzo Ando, tried to explain his motives to the Admiral, whom he admired. Suzuki cut him and said, 'If that's all you have to say, then shoot'. Ando then shot him, but not fatally. Suzuki's wife rushed in and outfaced the assassins with her own courage. I was impressed by Suzuki's calm indifference to death.

But the big surprise came soon after the war, when I met postal minister Hisatsune Sakomizu, who had been cabinet secretary at the end of the war under Suzuki, who was then prime minister. Sakomizu gave me a lunch in private and presented to me a copy of his book about the concluding stages of the war, adding some personal comments. He said that the old premier seemed to do nothing, just reading and signing the papers which Sakomizu as cabinet secretary had prepared. 'I felt I was running the country', said Sakomizu. The old man just sat there reading *Tao-te Ching* by Lao-tzu, occasionally saying, 'Hot day, isn't it?'

But then one morning, Suzuki did not appear. The cabinet secretary, generally so cool and efficient, suddenly found that he could hardly do any work. He could not decide things; he found his hands shaking. He suddenly realized the terrible dangers which they were all running. And then when Suzuki came back in the afternoon, the atmosphere again became calm and resolute.

I have sometimes told this to Western people; they agree that we have nothing quite like it. To the West, Budo has associations with films of what we call blood-and-thunder. I believe that the deeper tradition of Budo calm should be known also. Japanese should get to know some of the incidents where it has been shown both in historical and modern times.

The Spirit of Budo

2

Old Traditions Breathe Fire into Present-day Life

The Spirit of Budo

Chivalry and Budo

The future of Budo is something which must come from Japanese themselves. No foreigner can decide it for them; nor can any single Japanese decide it. It must come from the inner life of the Budo tradition. But sometimes the interest shown by foreigners can help to reawaken interest in Budo among Japanese themselves.

Furthermore, to see how other countries have developed— or have failed to develop—their own traditions can be a hint for Japanese. I will now take the example of how the Western ideal of chivalry changed as it led to the ideal of the English gentleman. Chivalry developed among the European knights, especially the Normans, who brought it to Britain. It taught not only the ancient Roman virtue of bravery but also kindness to the weak, especially women, and respect for defeated enemies. The respect for the defeated was a big advance on the Roman idea: Romans were merciless. Their famous slogan was *Vae victis!* or 'Woe to the vanquished!' (It must be admitted that in actual war the knights often relapsed into the Roman way.)

The Norman chivalry was for a long time taught only among knightly families. Later it was gradually extended to 'gentlemen'. They were a grade below the knights but had to be from a good wealthy family.

The common people were not taught chivalry and knew it only from popular songs and romantic epics. They were not expected to practise it. Shakespeare for instance despised what he called the 'mob', that is, the common people. *Julius Caesar* begins with these lines about the common people: 'You blocks, you stones, you worse than senseless things!'

A Fifth Dimension of Chivalry

By Shakespeare's time, the 16th century, a new idea was coming up. A big change had begun in 15th century England. (Perhaps Shakespeare himself was an example: he was at first despised because his father had not had the money to send him to a university. Yet he became famous in his lifetime.) The enormously popular poet Geoffrey Chaucer declared that a gentleman is to be known by his good behaviour, not by his birth. A man is a gentleman, proclaimed Chaucer, only if he behaves well.

There was a verse of that time: 'There are these four virtues—Honesty, Kindness, Freedom and Courage. No one can be a gentleman if he lacks three of them'.

In other words, he must have at least two. It is typical of the British that this ideal does not require one to have more than two of the four virtues to be considered a gentleman. Of course, it is better if he has three—better still if he has four. But we do not expect such perfection to be common. (I am reminded of a phrase in a letter of Yamaoka Tesshu[9]: 'Every man has seven bad points'.)

I may add here that the virtue of freedom has been an enormous advantage to us in national life. We respect the freedom of others to be eccentric. To be eccentric is often a sign of genius. But in many countries, eccentric people are disliked and persecuted. The British respect for freedom is one reason why for centuries there have been many new ideas arising in Britain.

However, even when complete, the ideal has some big gaps in it. Nothing is said about inner calm. Courage included endurance of pain. This was especially a Roman virtue. At school we learnt how Scaevola, a Roman hero captured by the Etruscan enemies about 500 B.C., was brought for interrogation. There happened to be a fire in the room. One of them said, 'Answer our questions'. Scaevola walked to the fire and thrust his right hand into it. The interrogators watched in amazement as the hand blackened and shrivelled. Then he faced them and said, 'Ask'.

It is pleasant to read that the Etruscans freed him and allowed him to return to Rome. (Romans would not have been so chivalrous.) The Romans honoured him by giving him the name 'Left-handed'; *Scaevola* means left-handed. His descendants played a large part in Roman history for six centuries. Some of us schoolboys were impressed by this. When I read about Nobunaga's death[10], dancing in the burning temple, I said to myself, 'Scaevola!'

This sort of grand-scale heroism is outside ordinary life. But there were also small-scale incidents in the tales of chivalry which could be tried. As a boy I read how a Knight and his servant were travelling and stayed at a poor inn, where the beds were full of fleas. 'The servant was scratching all night, but the Knight lay still'.

On one occasion, when my family were on holiday, we were overtaken by a storm and had to stay at a little inn. My bed had fleas in it. I resolved to imitate the Knight, trying to lie still and letting them bite. After two or three bites, they stopped and I began to fall asleep. Then I felt a new bite and automatically scratched. I concluded that the Knight in the story must have stayed awake.

As a student at London University, I joined a Spartan-type group. Once a week, we bathed in the icy water of a deep pond; it was a special achievement to break the ice in winter months. About this time I began Judo and heard from the old teacher that the traditional samurai always washed his face in cold water, 'so that it would remain firm even after death'. From then on for over 20 years I never took a hot bath. I used hot water only reluctantly just to shave.

But there was a gap in the code of chivalry: there was no inner calm. The Knights were passionate people. The gap was filled in the 19th century by reviving the Roman virtue of inner undisturbability, not merely outer calm. The nation as a whole began to cultivate it. There was a familiar saying on the Continent: 'the calm Englishman'. Anti-British writers, like the popular novelist Jules Verne, often laughed at the British for stupidity, but admitted that they were calm.

The Emerging Ideal of Budo

There was, however, another big gap in the gentleman ideal, which was never filled. I realized this gap for the first time when I went to Japan. Our list of virtues—Honesty, Kindness, Freedom, Courage and also

Calm—says nothing about culture at all. This compares very unfavourably with the Japanese tradition. Of course, not all the Japanese warriors were cultured. But they were ashamed if they did not have some culture, and they respected culture in others, whereas in Britain the gentleman did not feel ashamed even if he had almost no knowledge of literature or music.

True, a few refinements in behaviour were expected of him and his wife. But the ideal was fine character and especially self-control, and not culture. There were indeed many highly cultured and intelligent gentlemen. But culture and intelligence (dare I say it?) were regarded as extras, so to speak. They were desirable, but not essential.

There was, and still is, a criticism: 'He is too clever'. No Frenchman would make such a criticism; he would never think one could be too clever. But the English word 'clever' corresponds to 'zuru-gashikoi'. We both associate extreme cleverness with cunning.

There was even a view that too much culture could be somehow weakening. For instance, a general who was also a poet might be regarded with suspicion. General Wavell, later Viceroy of India, published a book of poems. But they were not his own; his book was an anthology, called *Other Men's Flowers*. It used to be said that if a soldier wanted to publish poems, he did it under a woman's name.

Perhaps this attitude has begun to change now. There is more poetry in the newspapers, magazines and on the radio. Changes in Britain are very slow, but it may be that the ideal gentleman will have to practise some form of culture. In the last 40 years, the whole concept of the gentleman has been under attack from socialist egalitarians. But socialism has been a disastrous failure all over the world. It failed in the fields where it claimed to be strongest: economic organization, scientific advance, education and freedom. So the gentleman ideal may have a strong revival. But it cannot be revived in its past form: it must find new forms.

In the same way, I believe, the Budo ideal too is beginning to find new forms. In the little history which I have given above, the gentleman ideal found new life in the 19th century by reviving the old Roman idea of inner calm, not merely outward stoicism. So too, I am sure, the new forms of Budo will incorporate elements which were there in its past, but which did not come to flower.

World Culture and Budo

To a few foreigners, Japan is a second home. I am excluding the sentimentalists who are fascinated by the polite surfaces of Japanese life. Most of them are living comfortably sheltered from its deeper realities. Usually they can neither read a Japanese magazine or book nor speak more than broken sentences. These people are not at home in Japan, though they sometimes think they are. They are more like guests.

Home is a place not only of security and affection, but of quarrels and struggles. Furthermore, it is a place where in the middle of the quarrels and struggles we give—and find—love. In spite of all the faults, we want to be there. A few foreigners can feel that about Japan. They know all the defects, but still want to be there: it is home.

For still fewer of us, it is a sort of third home. We are the ones who lived in Japan in 1940 and again in postwar Japan. Britain has not changed so much: Japan has changed completely. Or so it seems, but has it?

I am often asked, 'How much has Japan changed?' If it is English people who are asking, I often say, 'When you get home from work, what is the first thing you do?' 'I usually change', they answer, meaning that they take off their working clothes, whether factory or office, and change into their comfortable home clothes. In English this is called 'changing'. And I will tell them, 'Well, that is how Japan changes'.

Different Patterns of Behaviour

This does not mean that Japan is insincere. But there are certain attitudes—ways of thinking, ways of behaving, which are appropriate in one environment. But in a different environment, others are more appropriate. The clothes, so to speak, change. The man or woman changes them, but the person remains the same underneath the changes.

To some extent, this is true of all nations. Talking to foreigners, a Frenchman feels that they expect him to say something witty or clever. (Some Frenchmen admit that they prepare a few witty remarks in advance.) An Italian is expected to be charming. (Some of them say it is very tiring.) These are the clothes which they wear. Sometimes they take their coat off; then the foreigner gets a shock.

A political quarrel in France can descend to personal insults which would never be tolerated in Britain, and the Italian Mafia is not charming. But still, though the clothes are only clothes, they do in fact reflect something of the nature of those who wear them. The Italians charmed the world with music, as we see from all those Italian words like allegro, piano, sonata and hundreds of others.

Though an English Savile Row suit and a first-class Italian suit do have many points in common, they are not the same. A typical Englishman wearing a good Italian-made suit does look well-dressed. But somehow he lacks the dashing air which the suit seems to need. Similarly a typical Italian in a Savile Row suit somehow misses the unselfconscious dignity. The clothes in both cases are largely the same, but there is a difference of style, and the foreigner often is not fully at ease in that style.

I sometimes have the impression that Japanese are wearing foreign designs of behaviour. They wear them very well, but there is something not quite natural about them. And this is because those patterns of behaviour have not been developed from Japan itself. But there are one or two exceptions where Japan has been spectacularly successful in developing a new adaptation—a new style of an accepted behaviour pattern.

One such example is industrial capitalism. In the earlier days of Japan's industrialization, it was as ruthless as the Western model: in 1940 a friend told me how the workmen in his father's factory had worked all day and slept under the machine at night. Japan gradually changed such practices, but they did not simply reform. They introduced entirely new concepts of management relations, almost undreamt of in the West.

When I lecture on Japan, I can amaze the audience by quoting the president of one of the largest electrical companies, who announced an extra bonus with these words:

'I am glad you are going to get this extra. I know some of you are short of money. But it will not make you happy, because soon you will increase your commitments, and you will be just as short of money as before. So you will be no happier. But what will make you happy is to know that you are making good-quality, reliable and cheap electrical appliances for the Japanese housewife. That will make you happy, and nothing else will'.

No Western company president would talk like that. He might talk of the good reputation of the company, which would make it successful and so benefit everyone in it. But he would not talk about happiness. That would be a private matter for each employee. A good management would make the company successful and give increasingly good wages and conditions for the staff. But how they use these advantages—whether they were happy or not—would be entirely for each individual and has nothing to do with management.

I once asked Shigeo Horie, then president of the Bank of Tokyo, whom I had known rather well for over 20 years, whether he felt responsible for the happiness of his staff. He replied: 'Yes. Without any qualifications or reservations, yes'. I then asked Kiyoshi Hara, then president of Asahi Broadcasting Company, the same question. 'Yes. I don't expect that I shall always succeed', said he, 'but... yes, I do feel responsible'.

I must add also that both these two remarkable men expected their staff to be prepared to work very long hours, if necessary. They themselves did so during crises.

Once, when president Hara was having dinner with me, I noticed that he was very tired. I expected that after dinner he would go home to bed. To my surprise, he remarked that afterwards he would go to the airport to greet one of their TV teams which had just achieved a big success in Beijing. A Western company president would never do such a thing. The TV team would be exhausted and should be given the chance to rest. The next day they would be given a big welcome at the broadcasting station. In this Japanese case, the president himself was also exhausted. Still both sides would recognize the value of this personal greeting. Their very tiredness would make it all the greater.

How Budo Contributes to World Culture

We recognize the Budo spirit of rising above the tiredness of body. We see it again, on a much deeper level, in the independence of money grabbing among many ordinary Japanese. In Britain we are used to giving tips for good service; we have always been surprised when Japanese refused them. (Perhaps recently we have begun to corrupt them.)

But it surprises us when we see that this same spirit of independence and honesty does not extend to politics. In Britain we have financial scandals, but they never involve politicians. In the fiercely fought election campaign of 1992, there were many personal attacks on politicians from the other side and from newspapers. But there was not one accusation of financial dishonesty. I would guess that this is one of the new fields where the Budo spirit will show itself.

The purification of politics is not at all impossible. In the last century, British politics was hopelessly dishonest and corrupt. We can read vivid descriptions of it in Dickens.

In 1892 London was run by the Metropolitan Board, which was famous for dishonesty. When it was proved that a director of the Board had taken a large sum of money from a builder, he maintained that it had been just a friendly gift, and that he had done nothing in return. There was a famous cartoon which showed this director as a baby in the cradle with hard-faced businessmen dropping golden coins into the cradle. The caption said, 'He never did anything for it: it was always just a friendly gift!'

In general the ruthless businessman was admired. It was he who built railways, roads, houses and great bridges all over the world like the huge one at Calcutta. He brought prosperity to the country. If he was dishonest, well....

Darwinian evolution, understood by nonscientists to be simply 'survival of the fittest', supported the idea that the weak and stupid and lazy must simply perish. The Church was defenceless against these ideals. Little girls of six were employed in factories for tiny wages: they soon died, but others took their place. The businessman felt he must be hard. In some offices, spectacles were forbidden; they were regarded as a sign of weakness. Some hard men refused the new anaesthetics before an amputation. (My own uncle, who was in the Royal Navy, had to have a toe cut off: he refused to have ether.)

These merciless entrepreneurs were not gentlemen. The gentlemanly ideals of fairness and compassion were preserved in the countryside among landowners. Some of them were not rich: but whether rich or poor, they would not talk to the newly rich businessmen. The latter felt slighted and began to desire to become gentlemen. So they sent their sons to the small country schools, where the old ideals of the gentleman were still cultivated. As these sons grew up, the ideas of the men of wealth began to change. The figure of the perfect gentleman—calm, brave, quiet, honest and kind—was struggling to public consciousness.

In the course of time, the public view of political corruption began to change. Up to the end of the 19th century, the successful businessman or politician was admired, even if he was dishonest. In the 20th century any suspicion of financial dishonesty is a bar to a career as a politician. We have big financial scandals but no big political ones.

As an outsider, I wonder how the Budo spirit of Japan will struggle to the surface of Japanese life. After all, many samurai—like British country gentlemen—were poor compared with the traders. It is not something which even a Japanese could consciously plan: it must rise from the depths of the spirit. But I hope it will not be the Budo of yang—swaggering, bullying, mindlessly aggressive and narrow. That would lead to isolation and ultimate ruin. I have faith in Japan and believe that it will be the Budo of yin—gentleness in strength, strength in gentleness, associated especially with culture. I believe this can be Japan's contribution to world culture.

Britain gave the gentleman ideal to the world and we are proud of having done so. But there is a big gap in it. The gentleman, it has been remarked, can be a bit boring, if he has no sense of humour and no appreciation of art. Of course, many gentlemen have a good sense of humour and appreciation of art. But it is not formally part of the ideal. One can be a good gentleman without either.

The Japanese ideal of *bunbu ryodo,* or the pen and the sword, thus supplies something missing. Of course, Japan cannot simply revive this old slogan: it can, and must, take a new form. But I think this will be one of Japan's real contributions to the advancement of world culture. Only when that contribution is made, will Japanese feel at peace within themselves.

Impulsive Generosity

One of the most attractive features of the Japanese character is a sudden, uncalculating impulse of generosity. Much of the kindness in Britain is based on religion or a feeling for social justice. They are part of a lifestyle: the individual case is just part of that plan of life. But in Japan these actions are not based on any grand principle: they are spontaneous. (Of course in Japan, there is also the organized charity of religion and social justice.)

To us, the sudden gesture of kindness seems to be somehow childlike. I do not mean 'childish'; I mean that it has the straightforwardness and total commitment of a child. A famous psychologist has remarked, 'It is only children who know how to give'. He explained that the adult people have always some anticipation or expectation of something in return for their gift. Or they give grudgingly, thinking of something else which they could have done with the money. 'Such reservations may be unconscious', he said, 'but they are still there'. Only children can give without any reservations.

Looking back, I can find an example of this in my own life. When I was nine years old, a speaker came to our school and told us about the great Tokyo earthquake. He showed us some terrible pictures, and his talk had a big effect on many of us. After the talk, the headmaster distributed little cardboard savings boxes to each of us. We were told that if we handed them in after a month, what we had saved would be sent to help the victims of the earthquake. The headmaster explained that we should not just feel sorry but we should do something.

We children had no money of our own, except sixpence a week to buy sweets. If we did some job in the garden, father would give us a penny or two. So for the next month, I and my next brother, aged 10, undertook a number of jobs. We put every penny we had into the two little boxes. My mother told us that we should keep a little for ourselves, but we did not do so. We had no sweets for a month. My mother respected our decision and did not give us any herself. I think she was pleased to see a strong decision.

But my eldest brother, aged 12, did not put in more than a little. He was already saving towards buying a bicycle. There was a target: when he had reached that, the parents had promised to give the rest. Most of the bigger boys of 13 did not give anything. They were fully taken up with their own affairs. I heard them talking, and some of them said: 'The little we could give will not make any difference in Tokyo. But it will make a difference to ourselves here'. They had already moved from the purehearted generosity of the child to the selfish calculations of the grown-up.

The Unforgettable Friend I Met Only Once

Still, there are some who can keep the child alive in themselves. I met one such person when I first took a Judo contest in Japan. I had trained hard in Britain, but of course we were limited to what we could learn from the old Japanese teachers there and occasional high-grade Japanese players. I was fairly strong at *harai-goshi* and *osoto-gari*. On the other hand, I had never met a really fast *kouchi-gari*. As it happened, this first opponent was skilled in it. I was totally unprepared for his attack and lost the contest in a few seconds. I was knocked out of the tournament at once.

The winners of contests then were given a little medal, a fact which I did not know. As I came out of the changing room into the crowd, someone caught my arm, pressed a little box into my hand and hurried away. Bewildered, I opened the box and found a small medal. I realized later that this must have been from my victorious opponent. He must have realized how depressing it would have been for me, and he gave me his medal.

Such a thing would be inconceivable in Britain. We too would feel sympathetic, but we would probably just say, 'Well, you had bad luck this time, but... .' Words are cheap and soon forgotten. But I still remember that gesture of friendship from a Japanese who met me only once and whom I never saw again.

If by any chance he reads this essay, I should like him to accept my 'Thank you'. I could not say it at the time, because I did not realize what had happened until after he had gone.

Another surprise came when I was watching one of the big tournaments. They did not have championships then, but we had the *senmon-bu* contests which were comparable to championships. In those days there was no *waza-ari* or *yusei-gachi,* so a contest was either won by *ippon* or was a draw. There were many draws, in which the result was decided by *chusen* or drawing lots.

On one occasion, a man (I will call him A) had got to the quarterfinal by winning three *chusen* draws in succession. His opponent had got there by winning three contests with *ippon*. They fought their contest, and the result was a draw. Accordingly, they were called to the side of the tatami to make the draw. But now A refused. A friend of mine who was standing near told me that A said:

'I give up the contest. He has won. I have been lucky three times, but he has scored *ippon* three times. Even if I were lucky again, I should be ashamed to beat a better man by luck'. And he withdrew.

'Is He a True Sportsman?'

I have never heard of such a thing in the West. Sometimes in all sports contests one man wins by amazing luck against a clearly better man. But that is accepted. It is simply part of life. Even a very strict sportsman would accept it and not feel that he must try to change a result. In this Judo tournament, an English sportsman would probably think: 'After all, I drew with him in our contest. His previous wins may have been against weaker opponents than I met'.

Of course, there may be difficult decisions in sportsmanship. As a student I became fairly strong at chess and in later years I was in the BBC team. Every year the British champion gave a simultaneous exhibition against about 20 BBC players. I had the satisfaction of drawing against him four times. One of our team was a former Hungarian, now a naturalized Briton, whom I will call T. He was very strong at correspondence chess, in which moves were exchanged by letter. The players had one or two days to think between each move, so the games became very complicated. T became a member of the British team at that.

One year a correspondence team match was arranged between the British team and the Soviet team, then the strongest in the world. Every two days, a radio link was set up between Moscow and London, and the moves of the British team, or the Soviet team if it was their turn, were all sent together. T would decide his move and telephone it to the British end of the link. Then two days later, his Soviet opponent's reply would be read out to him.

One day, T said to me, 'I want your advice as an English sportsman'. I felt a bit embarrassed, but he went on: 'I've had a cable from my opponent in Moscow saying that his last move was a mistake. He wants to substitute a better one. Should I agree?'

To his evident surprise, I said: 'No, you and he are members of a team. He should be more careful. Go on, and win'.

'But is that sportsmanlike?' he asked. 'Poor fellow, he made a mistake'.

'Don't be sentimental', I said. 'He is a tough professional, probably. And he is not a sportsman. No true sportsman would ask such a thing'.

T looked disappointed in me. Perhaps he was wondering whether I really was an Englishman. He did allow the Moscow man to amend the move, and the game was a draw. From my point of view, T was simply sentimental. True sport means to try very hard and then to accept win or loss without being at all upset. In this way it is a good training for life.

But this is part of a pattern, and it is not spontaneous like the Japanese examples. Some say that such things do not happen today, but they do. I know that many Japanese are hard, scheming, ruthless, backbiting, like the rest of us humans. But occasionally the heart is lightened by seeing one of these independent acts, like a flower on a muckheap. In most countries people do not put flowers on top of a muckheap, but one can see it even today in Japan.

On Humour

When foreign people are asked to give a lightning impression of the British, many of them mention 'mania for dogs, the gentleman ideal, honesty in politics and something called a sense of humour'. Then they go on to give individual opinions. Frenchmen say that Englishmen are crude and cold, and I have heard Japanese call us *yabottai* (unrefined) and also cold. Russians wonder why the English are always complaining, like Russian farmers.

As to the dog mania, I admit that it is true. Often British people say to me: 'What are Japanese people really like? I have talked to some Japanese, and they were all very serious'.

'You forget that they had to use a foreign language to talk to you', I would tell them. 'They wanted to get their English sentences right—that is why they were serious. You would be serious if you had to talk to them in Japanese: they would be making jokes, and you would be silent'.

Then I go on to tell them about Hachiko[11] and the statue of Saigo with his dog. When they hear that, British people warm to the Japanese.

Now, however, I want to say something about the famous British sense of humour. Of course, individuals in every nation have it, but in Britain it is a national characteristic. Perhaps you will be surprised to hear that it is a form of bravery.

There are many kinds of bravery. But I believe that both Japanese and British respect calm bravery more than shouting swagger. The calm hero rises above the present danger: he meets it but without inner agitation. Wonderful! But the sense of humour adds something more to calm bravery: it finds laughter even in the danger or difficulty.

Life as a Laughing Matter

I will give an example. During the bombings of cities in World War II, citizens everywhere showed great courage. At the height of the bombing of London, some American newspapermen asked ordinary citizens of London about their feelings. One reporter said that he was amazed not only by the brave determination but by the cheerfulness of the Londoners.

One working man had told him that he was not at all afraid of being hit by a bomb. The man said: 'How can a German bomber kill me? First of all, he has to find London and then he has to find the East End of London. I live in Alton Street, Number 32. So he has to find Alton Street and then find Number 32. When he has found it, he has to drop his bomb on it. And even if he does, probably I'll be out, having a drink at the pub'. This ordinary Londoner could not only face the bombs but also laugh at them with this comical story.

In English we distinguish wit from humour. Wit is a clever way of saying something indirectly which cannot be said directly. It is often a way of attacking someone. The French are famous for it. The French writer Voltaire was shown a poem by a rival author, entitled *A Message to the Future*, and remarked, 'I doubt if this message will reach its destination'. In other words, no one will read the author's work after he is dead.

The French constantly make witty sarcastic remarks about their neighbours, the Belgians. After hearing one of these, I asked the Frenchman, 'Do the Belgians make sarcastic witty remarks about the French in return?' He looked at me. 'They would like to do that', he said, 'but they are Belgians, so they cannot think of any!'

We British can appreciate such wit, but most of us do not really like it. It is bitter. The farther east you go in Europe, the bitterer the wit becomes. The Hungarians say about themselves, 'If you have a Hungarian as your friend, you do not need an enemy'. In other words, you can never trust him. (I have not found this true in my own experience.)

Japanese people should know about these acid international jokes; such things are common. And there is no need to be sensitive when some are told about Japan. The Hungarians even invent slanders about themselves; so do Jewish people.

Sometimes the wit says something very interesting. Vasary Tartakower was a Hungarian cavalry officer at the beginning of this century. He was famous as a duelist. In those days duels were frequent, but they stopped as soon as blood came from the first wound. The wounded man lost the duel. After World War I, the Hungarian army ceased to exist. Tartakower entered university, took a doctorate and finally became a brilliant chess master, one of the best in the world.

Near the end of his life, he was interviewed by a journalist, who said to him, 'There must be very few people who have had so many triumphs'. Tartakower gave a little smile and said: 'I have never had a real triumph. Whether at dueling or at chess, I have never beaten a man who was wholly well!' He was hinting wittily that a loser always has an excuse.

What Budo Does Not Teach

The true sense of humour is entirely different from wit. It is almost never an attack on someone else. It consists in looking at one's own misfortune from above and finding something to laugh at in it. Budo teaches calm endurance, but humour teaches more than that.

I have visited some prisons in London and know what they are like. They are crowded. Britain has more people in prison proportionally than other European countries. On the other hand, there is less crime in Britain than in most other countries. I once read the memoirs of a former prisoner, who was sentenced to four years for burglary. He said that the food was very monotonous, and some of the prisoners appointed him their spokesman to complain to the governor. The governor was a just man and was respected. The prisoner saw him and stated the complaint.

'The prison food has been approved by the independent prison inspectors', said the governor. 'They confirm that it is well balanced and healthy. And I have exactly the same food myself here every day. I do not expect you to eat what I do not eat myself'. The prisoner looked at the governor's face and knew that it was true.

'Yes, but yours is cooked specially for you, isn't it? Ours is cooked by mass production'.

The governor replied seriously: 'Yes, probably mine is better cooked than yours and a bit more tasty. But after all, if you don't like prison food, why come to prison?' The prisoner said he could not help laughing. The governor laughed too, and the interview was ended.

In his memoirs the prisoner wrote: The governor's words— 'If you don't like prison food, why come to prison?'—were a great help to him then and also afterwards in life. He never offended again. If he was tempted, the phrase floated up from his memory: 'Why come to prison?' In his heart, he thanked the governor, who had used the sense of humour to awaken a sense of responsibility. The prison circumstances did not change, but they became bearable.

Even in very small things, humour can be a great help. Once a year my accountant comes to my house to make up my income tax accounts. He brings a little portable calculator, which makes a buzz as it prints. I must be in the same room, because he occasionally has a question. One day I sat on the other side of the room, trying to do an urgent piece of writing. It was very irritating to be constantly interrupted by the bzz-bzz of the little printer. The young accountant, a good friend of mine, realized this. He stopped for a moment and said, 'Every time this printer goes bzz, it means that you will pay less tax'. We both laughed. In a way it was ridiculous, but in fact I was no longer irritated by the bzz-bzz. The situation had not changed, but now I welcomed it.

A sense of humour is not part of the gentleman ideal, and as far as I know it is not part of Budo. But it is perhaps a very useful addition to those ideals. Here is a last example. When the Soviet space programme began, they sent up insects, then some rats, then dogs, and finally in 1961 Yuri Gagarin, the first man in space. It was arranged that Gagarin should make international tours. He was a handsome modest man, and crowds lined the streets in London to see him pass. He stood up in the car, and the people clapped and waved.

The then Prime Minister Harold Macmillan, with some of his friends, watched Gagarin pass. They remained quite calm outwardly, like gentlemen or *bujin*. But one of them murmured to Macmillan, 'This is a tremendous propaganda triumph for the Soviets'. 'No', replied Macmillan. 'And perhaps they have missed their chance in Britain. Thank Heaven! They did not send one of the dogs!'

Technical Training as a Means

When one looks at a high-speed photograph of a ballet dancer in mid-leap, one can get an uneasy feeling. One knows that this figure is not really flying and must come down very quickly. Yet it remains impossibly hanging in the air. It is very unnatural and against the whole spirit of ballet dancing, which is movement. The photograph is frozen movement: it is a contradiction. So it makes some people feel uncomfortable, and I am one of them.

Soon after I began Judo in 1930 at the age of 16, I had this kind of experience in connection with Budo. I was a member of the London Budokwai (yes, this is how it was spelt), the first Judo club in Europe. Every year we had a big public display, which was mainly Judo. I remember the exhibition of *ju no kata* (basic forms of Judo) by the two Japanese instructors—Gunji Koizumi, an art expert, and Yukio Tani, a full-time teacher. Tani had been very famous at the beginning of the century, as one of the few Japanese experts who introduced Judo and *jujutsu* to Europe, defeating wrestlers and boxers easily. They are mentioned in a Sherlock Holmes story and in Bernard Shaw's play *Major Barbara*.

I noticed that after one of the longest *ju no kata* movements, Tani gave what seemed to be a deep sigh. I watched him carefully and discovered that he held his breath for the whole duration of each of the movements. For a long time I felt too awed to ask him about it. Finally I did so, and he answered briefly, 'The *bujin* must keep fullness during the *waza*'. He never explained it further. His father and grandfather had been *jujutsu* masters, and he was evidently keeping to a tradition. I was suitably impressed. I felt—as most of us did—that everything Japanese had behind it a mysterious secret of great value.

Achieve the Freedom of Mind

But soon afterwards I had a big surprise. Besides the main Judo display, there used to be short demonstrations of other *bujutsu* arts. There were some Japanese Kendo men in London. Also at the first display I saw, there was a demonstration of the weight-and-sickle against a swordsman. Later in the programme, a Kendo man came up again, but this time faced an opponent armed with what looked like two round wooden plates with a handle at the back. They looked like very thick saucepan lids. With these he was able to parry the attacks by the sword and finally win by smothering the swordsman's arms and by hitting him on the face with one of the plates. There was no commentary, and the audience watched in bewildered silence—another Japanese mystery.

Afterwards I asked one of the senior members, who said that the plates were indeed supposed to represent saucepan lids. A famous fencing master, he said, had told his pupils that a true master was not dependent on having a sword. He told his pupils that they could attack him at any time, as a test. So one of them came at him with a sword, while the master was cooking in his kitchen. The master snatched up two saucepan lids, with which he parried the attack and finally subdued the pupil. Then the pupils began to study methods of using saucepan lids, and it became a school of technique.

Only my reverence for things Japanese prevented me from bursting out laughing. The whole point of the incident was to show that a true master could use anything. He must not be dependent on any particular thing. In this case, it happened to be saucepan lids. Tomorrow it would be something else; he would not have saucepan lids.

It seemed to me that the pupils had completely misunderstood. The point was to be able to pick up anything and use it effectively. But they froze at saucepan lids.

If we look at Budo classics, we can see that the masters were aware of this danger. Again and again they say: 'Technical training is the means to arrive at the state of freedom. When he has mastered the training, the training ceases to exist for him. This is the supreme aim of all the Ways'. We can find this in the *Heiho-kadensho* of about 1630, which says: 'Forgetting the training, throwing away all minding about it so that I myself have no idea about it—to reach that state is the peak of the Way. This state is to pass through training till it ceases to exist'.

My impression is that while the Japanese tradition is very strong in assiduous training, it is rather reluctant to 'give up training' at the very end. I will give an example from another field.

A Japanese who came to work in London for three years had a daughter remarkably talented in the piano. He asked me to help him find a good teacher. I knew that one of the best teachers, who had been internationally famous, was still alive. We managed to arrange for the girl to play to him. He was impressed and arranged for her to have lessons from one of his pupils. This was good luck, and the father was grateful.

A year later he told me that she was making good progress. But one day he came to me in some distress. 'I shall have to find another teacher for her', he told me.

'Why, what has happened?' I asked.

'He told my daughter at the last lesson to forget about playing the notes correctly and try to play purely as an expression of feeling'.

'They sometimes do this', I said. 'It is important to practise jumping beyond concentration on the notes alone'.

'It can't be right', he said, 'to tell her not to be careful about correct notes'.

'He is not saying that', I assured him. 'But one must be able to master them and then forget them'. He looked doubtful.

Jumping Beyond Skill

I found a clipping of an interview with M. L. Rostropovich, a world-famous cellist and conductor, in which he remarked: 'I would rather hear a cello piece played with genuine expression, even if there are two or three wrong notes, than a perfectly accurate but soulless performance'.

I also got a recording of Rostropovich conducting *Tosca*. This opera has no overture, begins with five great chords on the whole orchestra, and then the curtain goes up. The composer gives the tempo: the five chords are about three seconds each, so they continue for about 15 seconds. Then the opera begins. When he conducts this opera, Rostropovich thinks that the bare 15 seconds are too short. He makes the group of chords last nearly 40 seconds. 'I know this is not what the composer indicated', he says. 'But I believe it is more effective as an introduction to the great tragedy. It must be judged by the listeners'.

Of course, it is only some one with a mastery of music who can be so free. Sometimes young stage directors in Britain have tried to alter Shakespeare to make him appear a Communist or something like that. But they failed, because they were not masters of the theatre.

But it is important that when a good level of skill has been reached, one should make a jump beyond skill. Some Japanese teachers of English, who have a wonderful knowledge of the English language, are unwilling to make the jump. They still prepare their English sentences in their heads and then utter them. They want the sentences to be perfect, but the result is that they speak more correct English than Englishmen do. When we talk to them, we feel that we are talking to an English grammar book. Written English ought to be perfect, but spoken English is often very loose, like spoken Japanese.

For instance, recently I heard a government minister answer a question in Parliament. 'We can only help them if they apply', he said. What he meant was that the government can help people only if they apply for help; if they do not, the government can not know that they need it. The sentence was understood by the questioner and by everyone else. No one corrected him. But to express this meaning grammatically, the sentence should have been: 'We can help them, only if they apply'.

The rule is that 'only' is placed immediately before the word it qualifies. So in the actual statement, the minister is saying that if people apply, the government can 'only help', and that it cannot do more than help. This is the strict grammatical meaning.

This is a typical mistake in spoken English. But in fact everyone understood what the minister intended from the context. We expect such minor mistakes. If someone had corrected him, the minister would have laughed and then apologized, saying, 'I will take more care in the future'. And everyone else would have laughed too.

So we can come back to the saucepan lids. The master used the saucepan lids to defend himself successfully. It is true that the later technical experts in saucepan lids might be even more skilful in using them. But that is not the point. If they attained great skill in saucepan lids, they would still have no more than that: without saucepan lids their skill would be nowhere. But the Budo master would be able to use the *hibashi* charcoal tongs or anything else, or even nothing else.

The Spirit of Budo

3
Budo: Learning for Life

The Spirit of Budo

Travel and Learn

In a small book of introduction to Budo entitled *Budo shoshin-shu,* there is a section called 'Shukke-shi,' in which Daidoji Yuzan[12], the author, says that samurai should travel round and learn while they are young, as do the Zen monks. This book points out that Buddhist monks are in general far more educated than most samurai. It is because the monks 'leave their homes: they leave their monasteries and make tours to visit other monasteries, where they study various other doctrines and also get to know other regions'.

The author also says that many samurai just stay at home and draw their salary, without learning anything new except the place where they live. He recommends that samurai, like monks, should travel in order to learn and travel alone as the monks do. Really he is recommending something like a *musha-shugyo* errantry, not to study swordsmanship but to see new things and people with his own eyes. In this

way he will get not more book knowledge but judgement and will be able to judge what he reads.

The same idea would be good today. In Daidoji Yuzan's time, Japanese people could not travel abroad. Today they are wonderfully well informed through books. Even when they travel abroad, they go in groups, so that they are still at home in 'a little traveling Japan'. They look at the foreign country as if through a pane of glass.

They see us, turn to their friends on their side of the glass and talk about us. They do not talk to us face to face: they are always in a group with a glass plate round them. If they talk, they talk through the glass. They know so much, yet they act as if they knew very little.

Going Alone

In fact, the Japanese have so much theoretical knowledge that sometimes they cannot easily make a decision. Of course, if a road branches into two, it is easy to make a decision: you go either right or left. But if it branches into five roads, it is far more difficult to choose. If it branches into 17, it may take a very long time to decide. Some Japanese feel that the safest thing to do is to choose a road which already has several people on it.

But that is not really a decision: it is a sort of panic. How can the Budo spirit help to make us decisive? Let us first look at the causes of the indecisiveness. I believe that the main causes of the difficulty are lack of judgement, lack of confidence and lack of faith.

Judgement cannot be developed by reading. Reading gives us only certain facts and opinions, but it does not tell us how to judge them. For instance, books and TV may tell us many conflicting things about human mental potentialities. Some say genetic factors set absolute limits. However, look at children in India doing mental arithmetic. The teacher has a calculator, calling out some long numbers to be added, while the children are supposed to write them down.

At the end he says: 'That's all. Now add them'. But before he can press his 'Add' button, several of the children have shouted the answer. They had kept a running total in their heads. (Their technique of adding is to begin with the millions.) All the children can do this, though some are slower. To see this once makes one realize that no one can set limits to mental possibilities. One can now judge, because one has a living personal experience.

Someone may say, 'Oh, we could see that on TV'. Not so. An individual, sitting quietly in a corner, can see it happen. But a group or a TV camera would disturb the class. The children would be shy and not shout out the answer. So the group would see nothing. True, it might be rehearsed for TV, but then it would be no evidence at all: it is not a real happening but a stage show.

A traveller can get real experience when he is alone. Even just two foreigners together, talking their own language quietly, are still noticeable. The local people may adapt their behaviour, more or less. But a single person, not talking, is just a member of the public. He has read about French courtesy and he can look at the wonders of Paris. But now he can also see two Frenchmen quarreling. As one Frenchman remarked, 'We French civilized Europe, but perhaps we did not quite finish the job on ourselves'.

To see these things, we must practise going alone. The Budo text says, 'Do not forget the spirit of contest'. Many other texts say the same thing: 'Be prepared at all times to fight. In the street, at a meal, even in the bath, be ready'. At these times, the *bujin* would often be alone. Today we do not normally have to be ready to fight, but we should be ready to be alone. It takes courage, and the old Budo texts can help to give that courage.

With Faith in Fellow Human Beings

Secondly, many Japanese lack confidence in themselves. Even when they are expert at something, they are frightened of making some small mistake. This is perhaps because there is in Japan a bad habit of laughing at a mistake. All nations do this, but Japanese seem to do it more than others. When a foreigner comes up to me in London and asks, 'Me from Hungary ... where Westminster?' I do not laugh at his baby English. I know that if I were in Hungary, I would speak baby Hungarian. I smile and point the way. He is not ashamed, and we both understand the situation.

But sometimes a Japanese, who has a wonderful knowledge of English, hesitates nervously before speaking. He feels he must prepare a good sentence in his head before he speaks it. His nervousness makes me uneasy too. His literary English is too good for a casual conversation. (I feel as though I am back at school talking to the headmaster.) If he makes a small mistake, I do not laugh at the one percent that is wrong but admire the 99 percent that is right. But his colleagues would laugh at the one-percent mistake and ignore the 99 percent that is right. And he himself feels embarrassed, thinking I am secretly laughing at him. As a matter of fact, I feel rather relieved. He has been talking better English than I talk.

The Spirit of Budo

In general, Japan has a good reputation in the world today. When Japanese go abroad, they can have confidence. I do not mean they should boast and brag or quarrel. There are some Japanese boasters, but it is often a sort of bluff. Daidoji Yuzan remarks that the boasters of his time often had no real achievements at all, and it can be the same today. I am speaking of quiet confidence, which is based on real achievements. Real achievements do not need high-pressure advertising.

Faith is the third element which Japanese lack today. I believe that the Budo spirit has to develop some elements which have not yet appeared clearly. Many of the old texts say, 'When you leave your gate, you should assume that enemies are waiting'. In other words, the world is hostile: be prepared to fight it. *Budo shoshin-shu* reminds us of *fubo-shobu,* often translated as 'do not forget the offensive spirit', but I don't believe this is right. The characters for *shobu* mean a contest and not 'military glory'. *Budo shoshin-shu* makes it clear that it is fools and bullies who start quarrels and fights: the true samurai is restrained. He will resist them and does not himself start fights. But he is always ready if there is one.

In 1730 there were vendettas and feuds, and the clans mostly hated each other. Today it is different, though we foreigners are still surprised by how much Kanto and Kansai compete with each other. Japan is now one of the safest countries in the world. When they go abroad or they must meet foreigners, most Japanese think of them as potentially hostile: 'When you leave your shore, assume that enemies are waiting'.

There is another current in the Budo spirit. It is the *mutoryu* idea: the master swordsman does not use his sword. He does not see others as potential enemies but as potential friends. Dr. Jigoro Kano does not use the word *teki* or enemy in his writings. In 1933 I heard him speak in London about *jita kyoei,* which he explained—in his beautiful English—as 'mutual aid and concession leading to mutual benefit'. One principle of Judo, he said, was to learn how to appeal to the true human spirit which is in everybody. He told us that when we meet people, we should try to see not the outward form or their mental attitude alone but their true human heart. That heart, he said, is the same in them as it is in you.

I was impressed by his words which I heard when I was 18. I was taught as a child in London to beware of strangers. 'Never speak to anyone unless you have been introduced to them'. This was the maxim from the 19th century, when London was a really dangerous place; women tried never to walk alone. Today it is safer, though not as safe as Tokyo. After hearing Dr. Kano, I got more faith in fellow human beings.

I went alone to live for a year in Germany and Czechoslovakia, and later lived in Japan and India. I went camping alone in the Himalayas. Somehow I had confidence that I would be able to meet the tribesmen. When I got to the mountain state of Tihri, by chance I met an official, who spoke of me to the Maharaja. The King was horrified and said, 'Some bandits will rob and kill him'. So they gave me a horse and a guide. Such experiences give faith in human beings all over the world.

The Spirit of Budo

The Four Keys to Learning

Many years at Judo—first as a student and then as an honorary teacher in London—have given me some valuable lessons for life. I discovered that one can learn in four main ways—instruction, observation, inference and personal experience. My conclusion is that to know something thoroughly one must learn it in all these four ways. This applies to life in general, but we can see it in a model from Budo. Budo practice in a *dojo* training hall is like doing an experiment in a laboratory. If the correct result is clearly confirmed, one can recognize the same principle everywhere outside the laboratory, though not in such a clear form.

For instance, the principle of gravity is demonstrated in a laboratory, inside a vacuum. In the vacuum, a thread falls at the same rate as a stone. This does not happen in the world outside because of air resistance. But the same pull of gravity is still there. Once we have seen it in the laboratory, we can recognize it everywhere. The autumn leaves, blown high by the wind, seem to contradict gravity, but still we know that gravity is working on them. In the same way, in our Budo training in the practice hall, we can discover principles for our life outside. The *dojo* is a sort of laboratory: one of the things we can discover is how to learn.

To learn something positive we need these four methods— instruction, observation, inference and experience. They are all necessary, but not for a negative: 'Don't do that!'

Training the Inner Self

Instruction: Learning through instruction consists mainly of hearing and reading. Some people say, 'Instruction is wrong; let students find out everything for themselves by experiment'. That idea is nonsense. How can we say to a student? 'Here are some copper, zinc, acid and wire. Now discover electric current! Geniuses like A. Volta, M. Faraday and James Clerk Maxwell took only about 200 years. Perhaps you can do it in an afternoon'. Clearly it would be impossible; he must have some instruction.

For a negative—'Don't do that!'—the instruction alone should be enough. Judo beginners are often told: 'Do not try to prevent yourself from being thrown by putting your arm out on to the tatami. It is dangerous. You may dislocate your elbow'. In life a similar instruction would be: 'Do not drive a car when you are drunk'. These instructions may be followed, or not followed, depending on the intelligence of the pupil and also on how much he respects the instructor.

For many people, such warnings alone are not enough. 'A hundred hearings are not like one seeing'. The instruction may have to be confirmed by other means of knowledge.

Observation: This is seeing what happens to others. If we see an elbow damaged in the *dojo,* or a drunken driver go into a tree, the instruction is confirmed.

Inference: We look at some tough but not too intelligent Judo men and see how many of them cannot straighten one of their elbows. Or we can read about the many police-court convictions for drunken driving. We infer that the instruction was not right.

Personal experience: If in spite of the instruction not to do so, observations of accidents to others and inference from the long-term effects, we still do these things, then we get personal experience. Our own elbows are dislocated, or we drive into trees.

It is sometimes said that 'we must learn by personal experience alone'. But this cannot always be possible. If we get drunk, drive the car and crash into a tree, it is a personal experience. But often we shall learn nothing from it, because we shall be dead.

The Four Keys to Learning

Therefore, with negative things, personal experience is not necessary. It is usually undesirable. The most intelligent learn—from instruction alone—not to make mistakes. The less intelligent need observation and inference before they are convinced. The stupidly obstinate have to undergo a disaster before they understand, but quite often it is then too late.

My generation is very opposed to taking drugs, even though we drink tea and coffee which are mild drugs. Sometimes young people say to me: 'It is unreasonable to condemn drugs, if you have never taken them yourself, because you do not know about them from personal experience. You say they have bad effects, but how do you know what the effects are? You have never taken them yourself, so you do not know what the experience is like'.

Elderly people often do not know how to answer this argument and become silent. But I reply, 'I do not have to jump into a cesspit to know what it would be like.' Then usually the young people become silent, or else hurriedly change the subject.

So with negative things it is best to be able to accept instruction, without waiting for observation, inference and personal experience. We can learn this fact in the *dojo*.

But with positive things it is the reverse. Instruction is merely a starting point. It must be deepened by observation, inference and finally personal experience. There is always a danger that instructions will be too detailed so that the pupil follows them mechanically. Such a pupil may become technically expert, but he is simply like a machine. He can carry out his programme, but he cannot meet anything unexpected. The Budo schools knew about this danger.

The teachers would give the main points but not all the details. The students had to work out the details themselves. One of the 'secret scrolls' of the *Shinno shintoryu*[13] school says:

'My own teacher used to explain a technique to us only roughly and then tell me: "You have the root. Now you have to train relentlessly, crushing the bone and flesh, for a long time, never forgetting that the basis of our training is mental". *Jujutsu* is *shinjutsu*, or the art of the heart'.

Again and again these old traditions emphasize this: a Way or *do* is not simply a collection of tricks or a sequence of correct moves. There must be something living in it, which comes from a much deeper level than thinking: 'Now I will do this. Now it is time to do that'.

A Source of Calm Courage

This applies in many fields, including speaking a foreign language. Japanese students tend to learn correct grammar and many sentences by heart. But often they have no fluency. They have to prepare each sentence inwardly before they speak it.

I have sometimes taught the Japanese language to British people, and I have been told that my methods are rather unusual. But often the students become interested. Take the word *shitsurei,* for example. I explain that this means roughly 'Excuse me', and tell the student, 'You say this when there is some little accident, whether it is your fault or not'.

The student nods yes, and I make him say the word two or three times. Then I tell him to stand up and walk past me, brushing against me. He does so, silently.

Then I say: 'You should have said "Shitsurei" automatically'. I make him do it several times more, saying 'Shitsurei!' or 'Ah, shitsurei!' each time, till it comes naturally.

When he comes for the next lesson, I do not greet him at the door. I have switched off the hall light so that the little hall is dim. I leave the door half shut, and just inside I put a little table, so that when the door is opened it will be knocked over. As I hear him come up, I call out, 'Come in! ' He pushes the door, knocks over the table and says, 'Oh, sorry!' or 'What's this?' As he stands puzzled, I say: 'You should say "Shitsurei". Now go out again'. I put the table back and he comes in and knocks it over again, but this time saying 'Shitsurei'. We repeat the whole process two or three times. Students have told me that, after this experience, whenever they spilt or dropped something, 'Shitsurei' came out of their mouths without their thinking about it. Sometimes their British friends were bewildered.

Of course, these examples are not directly from Budo. But Budo can help us to overcome embarrassment. I have always thought it strange that a young Judo student will keep trying, even though he is thrown all over the *dojo*. He is not embarrassed, and no one laughs at him. They admire him.

But in speaking a foreign language, the Japanese feel embarrassed when they make a mistake, and other Japanese laugh at them. We should think of speaking a foreign language as *randori* in a *dojo*. The Budo spirit does not give us technique, but it gives us calm courage. With it, we can soon master technique.

The Spirit of Budo

Dynamic Words

'Boys, be ambitious!' I came across these words recently. A British teacher working in Japan told me about these words, which he said has had a profound effect on Japanese youth. It made me wonder: 'Have there been words spoken by Japanese which have had a deep effect on my own life?' There have been such words indeed, but I realize that they have not been general maxims like 'Boys, be ambitious!' They were individual remarks which were said to me directly or which I overheard.

A few such words were spoken by Yukio Tani, my Judo teacher. I heard them when I was about 17, and they made a lasting impression, because I was very keen on Judo. Tani had a wonderful reputation. When I was taught by him, he was already over 50, but was still very skilful. Over 20 years before, my father had seen this small man defeating big boxers and wrestlers, apparently by magic. He was a sort of god to us, and his words made a great impression.

Up to the age of 15, I was interested only in music. I never took any exercise, so I was constantly getting ill. The doctor told me that I must build up a better constitution, and I began running every day. Then I came across Judo. Soon I was very keen and began training. Tani noticed this and gave me a few lessons. Encouraged, I used to begin practice at 6 p.m. and stay till the end at 9 p.m.

The Unforgettable Words of Tani

One evening, however, I felt very tired with a headache. At about seven, I picked up my towel and prepared to leave the *dojo*. Tani looked across and asked, 'Where are you going?' I replied, 'I feel tired and I've got a headache. I'll come tomorrow'.

Tani asked quietly: 'If a man rushes at you in the street with a hammer, waiting to kill you, can you say, "I feel tired and I've got a headache, so come back tomorrow"?' Then he turned away. His words were like a thunderbolt. I went back on to the mat and practised. After half an hour he said, 'All right, go home now'. Somehow I felt I did not want to. I went on practising, but he gave me a little push with a smile and repeated, 'Go now, go now'. This time I went.

Later in life, when I have promised to do something but then have been tired or sometimes even ill, I wanted to make an excuse. Tani's words would return to me: 'Can you say, "I feel tired and I've got a headache, so come back tomorrow"?' Then I was able to put aside the tiredness and carry out the promise.

Another comment Tani made was not addressed to me, but it had a great effect. In those days the Budokwai members were mostly beginners and very clumsy. There were a very few skilful men to be models. So members had the idea that in a throw like *ashi-harai* you simply knocked the opponent's legs away from under him. They had not much idea of *tsuri-komi,* though of course it was shown to them by the teachers. They often bruised themselves and their opponents too. Soon after I had joined, I saw one member bruise his toes badly against his opponent's shin. He gave a loud cry and sat down on the mat, holding his foot and rocking to and fro with the pain.

Most of the other members stopped practising and watched as Tani walked across. He looked at the toe and felt it gently, while the injured man was still giving little moans. 'Only bruised', said Tani. 'Get up and sit at the side'. But the man still sat there, his face screwed up in pain.

Tani looked at him with concern. 'Shall I call your mother?' he asked. The injured man turned scarlet with embarrassment and got up quickly, hobbling off the mat. Somehow I felt embarrassed too. I made up my mind that he would never say such a thing to me. I did get injuries but I did not make a sound. I felt I would rather have the pain than hear the words: 'Shall I call your mother?'

Later on in Judo I was in the general tradition of not making a fuss. It is much easier to endure silently when one knows that all the others do so too.

A Justifiable Remark?

But I remember one occasion when there was quite a test. As a tall man, I used *ashi-harai* a good deal. On one occasion I met a tall Japanese who also used it. It was a sort of *ashi-harai* battle. Then, we moved at the same moment very fast. The feet met in midair; one of my toes were broken and the toe nail splintered. During practice one does not feel such things very intensely. I knew I had been hurt, but I thought it would be just a bad knock. My opponent in fact was only bruised. We went on practising, but began to slip. Looking down, we saw that there was blood on the tatami, and looked at each other: 'Me or you?' Then I saw blood streaming from my toe.

We wrapped it up and went to a nearby hospital, where one of the surgeons treated all our Judo injuries. He was a Kendo man. At that time there were a few Kendo men who felt that Judo was relatively modern and not quite in the traditional Budo tradition.

I sometimes felt his treatment of the Judo was rather— well— direct. No false sympathy there. On this occasion, he had to pick out the splinters of nail from the smashed end of the toe. He did it with a pair of tweezers, fragment by fragment. By now the toe was really hurting, and this of course was worse still. I managed not to make a sound or move the foot. He looked up at me once or twice during the little operation. What was going through my head were the words, 'Shall I call your mother?' No, you are damned well not going to call my mother!

He finished fishing for splinters, set the toe and bandaged it. As I prepared to go, he leaned back with a half-smile and said: 'I should think that was extremely painful'. I stood up, and he gave a little nod of approval. I realized that I had passed, in his private book, as not merely a foreign Judo man but also as a proper Budo man.

Tani said one thing about which I have never made up my mind. In my early days at the Budokwai, I was a member of the team which had matches against Oxford and Cambridge Judo clubs. They had no black belts, so our team was limited to *kyu* grades also. Once I was the captain. I had just got a brown belt, or 1st *kyu* grade. It was a team of five, and the contests were a five-minute *nihon-shobu*.

In this event Cambridge had won two matches, and the Budokwai had won two. So my contest was crucial. I quickly won a first point and I thought, 'I must not risk a counter'. I did not attack seriously again and gave no opportunities to my opponent. I won, and the team won.

But Tani would not speak to me afterwards. During the car ride back to London, he said nothing to me at all. Only when we parted, he said, "Coward!" I have never made up my mind whether this remark was justified. I can see that in the long run, it is better to practise attacking, even though one may sometimes lose to a counter. But (this is my British feeling, I suppose) I was a member of a team; this was crucial to the team. If I had been a member of the team—and my captain had lost by attacking again when he had already won—I would have said he was a fool.

My policy today (another British compromise) is to take the risk when I am alone, but if I am in a team I think of the interests of the team first.

What would be the traditional view of Budo?

Free from Fixed Ideas

There are some things which we have always thought to be natural and correct. We have never imagined that they could be any other way. Such beliefs may last all our lives. We never examine them. We think, 'Of course, that is so'.

Part of the inner training of Budo is to overcome such unconscious bonds. It must apply not only in the training hall but to life in general. It does not mean to change our ideas just because they are old or traditional. But we have to learn to see clearly where our beliefs are too narrow. Sometimes it is only when we go abroad that we find that people can think in other ways. But we must be alone among the foreigners; if our own countrymen are there too, we shall support each other. Then our fixed ideas will not change.

The Budo principle is meant to apply in other fields too. So before giving the Judo example, I will give one from music.

What's Unique to Western Music

When I was a boy, I trained as a pianist. At age 15, I wanted to become a professional pianist, but my father would not agree. I was furious: I gave up music and took up Judo instead. Still, I can say that I knew about Western music. But when I first went to Japan, I had a surprise. I got to know an old Japanese lady, who had two daughters. Both played the piano, and when I went to their house, they invited me to play the piano. She would listen to that without saying anything.

Sometimes they put on a gramophone record of an orchestra. Usually then the mother would go out of the room. I asked her once, 'Don't you like the Western music?' 'I don't like the orchestra music', she said. 'It is all so high up: *i-i-i-i-i-i-i*'. And she waved a hand high above her head. How ridiculous! But later, I thought about her remark. For the first time I realized that indeed most Western music has the melody high.

Our famous women opera singers are sopranos, who sing mainly at least an octave above middle C. On a violin only the lowest string can sound a middle C. It is true that the orchestra has cellos which play deep notes. But they rarely have the melody. On the piano, most notes of the melody are played by the little finger of the right hand, which sounds the highest note. Pianists have a very strong right-hand little finger. They can rest the hand on a table and hit it strongly with the little finger without moving the others. It makes a powerful rap.

The Japanese lady was right. I had never noticed that

Western music is high. And curiously, the older a classical composer became, the higher his music became. It is clearly heard in later Beethoven and Wagner.

Still, her remark did not make me change my appreciation of Western music. Unlike children's beliefs, the fixed idea had been reinforced by long practice and gone very deep. Theoretically I recognized that she was right. Western orchestral music has slipped higher and higher up the scale and is unbalanced. But it did not lessen my appreciation. When I went to live in India, I became interested in Indian music, which is in a lower register. (In Japan I was always so occupied with Judo, the Japanese language and Zen Buddhism that I had no time to learn any Japanese music.)

Physical training of Budo tries to get rid of the limiting habits we are born with. A strongly right-handed or right-footed man must develop both sides. Similarly, the inner Budo training must overcome inner habits, for instance, of always being on the attack or always defending and waiting to counter. The compulsive attacker must learn to wait; the compulsive defender must learn how to be a whirlwind.

This principle of learning is hinted at in many of the old Budo traditions. The serene warrior of yin must be able to imitate the raging warrior of yang, though remaining inwardly calm.

Emptiness and Fullness

When I taught advanced Judo classes at the London Budokwai, I sometimes used a special training method, based on this Budo principle. About halfway I divided the class, usually of about 60, into two groups—A and B. Then

I set them in pairs of roughly equal ability. I told the men in Group A: 'Practise as you would normally. Attack or be cautious, just as you like'. Then I said to the men in Group B: 'You must not make any attack or counter, till I call "Now!" You may defend yourself, but you must not attack or counter'.

'But when I call "Now!" you must attack continuously, without any break at all. You must go on, whether there's an opportunity or not, till I call "Stop!" If you're thrown, grab his foot from the ground and give it a pull, jump up and go at him without waiting to take a proper hold. Go mad in attack, till you hear "Stop!"'

Then I would call 'Begin!' Group A practised normally, making occasional attacks, while Group B just defended. They were hot and excited by the previous hour's practice. But now they must not attack. After about 30 seconds I could see some of them becoming impatient. They stole a quick glance at me to see if I had fallen asleep. But sometimes I kept silent for three minutes or more. Then I'd shout 'Now!' and they would jump furiously at the other man. In spite of their impatience, some of them found it difficult at first to keep up volleys of attacks for even half a minute. But finally most of them mastered it.

One might think that while this is fine training for Group B, it is not good for Group A, which knows after all that the opponent is not allowed to attack. But in fact, it is very good training for Group A too. It is true that the opponent is not now attacking or countering, but at any instant there may be the shout 'Now!' And then that same opponent will explode. It is like practising with a time bomb: it is quiet now, but it may go off at any moment.

Later on in the afternoon I would do the same practice, with Group A and Group B exchanging their places.

At the end of the two-hour practice, we used to sit in *mokuso* meditation for a few minutes, dripping with sweat. Afterwards I used to give a five-minute talk about the principle of the practice: 'Don't think that you are by nature an attacker, or by nature a defender. There is something in you which can be either. There's an old Budo saying "I have no strategy. I make *kyojitsu* (emptiness and fullness) my strategy". Emptiness means "not acting", and fullness "going into action". You must have both equally'.

Judo is meant to teach us this for life. Don't think 'My line is wait-and-see' or 'My line is to make things happen'. There is something in you which can do either, and Judo will help us to develop it.

Many years later, former members of that class told me that the practice was a great help to them. For instance, one man became a scholar and finally the head of a very important British library of rare documents. (The city records in London go back unbroken for 1,000 years and is unique in the world.) This man got to 1st dan and attended my black belt classes. Years later he told me how the Judo training helped him:

> I am a scholar, and I suppose that I am a quiet type of man. I don't like furious arguments. But occasionally we used to get visitors to the library who were aggressive and insisted on special treatment. They would not wait their turn, but demanded to go to the head of the queue.

If one became too noisy, the head of the library had to go down to see him. That was myself. On one occasion, a staff member came to me and said, 'I think this man is half mad: he looks as if he might attack us'.

So I went to see him. He did indeed look unbalanced. His face was red with fury, and he was dribbling at the mouth. He looked really dangerous, as if he were going to explode. I did not like the look of him, but as I went towards him, an extraordinary thing happened. 'I know this', I said to myself. 'I've been here before. I've been a Group A man, facing a Group B man who might explode any moment. Well, go on and explode! I don't care a damn for you or what you may do'.

And in fact he very quickly calmed down. He accepted that he must wait, even though he was a famous scholar from a famous foreign university. The story got around, and it gave me a good reputation with my staff and with regular visitors to the library. I owe it to the experiences in the Judo training classes.

The Spirit of Budo

4

Dr. Jigoro Kano and Judo

A lecture delivered at a meeting
of the British Judo Federation

The Spirit of Budo

The Buddhist Ideal of Mutual Benefit

When I was a boy, I heard Dr. Jigoro Kano speak in London. He was then 70, my age now. I thought he was a remarkable old boy, but I wasn't very impressed with remarkable old boys then, so I don't expect anyone to be impressed now.

His complete works, his complete writings, have just been published in Japan, and I telexed to have them sent by airmail. There are about 1,200 pages here in these three volumes, written in the old style of Japanese. I will just read you one little extract about Judo and other sports. Of course, things change, but this was the opinion of Dr. Kano, the founder of Judo. What I have here is a rough translation of the summarizing part of a short article which he wrote in 1929.

What We Learn from Judo

Recently competitive sports have become popular in Japan, and often the question comes up as to the relation between competitive sports and Judo. The question is put in various forms, but I will present the two extremes.

(1) There are those who attack competitive sports and say that since in Japan we have our martial arts (*bujutsu*) which are excellent for either spiritual education or physical education, or both, so what necessity is there for all the problems which will be involved in becoming enthusiastic to import sports? If we practise our own indigenous *bujutsu* arts, then we shall be encouraging the spirit of the Japanese people in a natural

way, and it will also be a training in virtue. But the import of foreign sports will naturally affect the spirit too, and perhaps we should end up as foreigners.

(2) Then again there are others who point to the good aspects of sports and say that Judo itself should be popularized as a form of competitive sports, and that it must be completely reduced in its practice to a form of contest, like sports of other kinds.

Neither of these ideas is correct, and one can suspect that each of the two sides has set out with some definite assumptions of what the relation between Judo and other sports ought to be.

As I have often explained, Judo is a Way which has a great universality. In the variety of its application, there are many different aspects from the point of view of martial arts, or physical education, or cultivation of intelligence and virtue, and also methods of application in daily life. Competitive sport is a kind of sport where it is a struggle for victory, and by that alone there is a natural training of the physical body. It is also a system of moral culture. If competitive sport is pursued correctly along these lines, it does have a great effect in physical and psychological training, and there is no quarrel about that.

But that object of competitive sport is a simple and narrow one, whereas the objective of Judo is complex and wide. Competitive sport pursues only one part of the objective of Judo. Of course, Judo can be treated simply as a competitive sport, and it may be all right to do so. But the ultimate objective of Judo cannot be attained in that way. So while we recognize that there is a demand these days to treat Judo on the lines of a competitive sport, on the other hand we must not forget what the real essence of Judo is and where it lies.

In these books of Dr. Kano, the same point comes up again and again. A competitive sport is something apart from our lives. We become experts, say, at tennis and then we are simply expert tennis players. It does improve the physical health, but that is where it stops. It has no application in our lives. But Dr. Kano based his principles of Judo on the idea of a method of learning something for life. It has been said that there are no rehearsals for life: You are on the stage *now*! But Dr. Kano thought of Judo as a sort of rehearsal, a way of learning things for our lives.

The Buddhist Ideal of Mutual Benefit

'Study for Yourself, Cultivate Yourself'

One basic principle which he put forward came from Buddhism—*Jita kyoei* or 'mutual benefit for oneself and others'. We in the West do not think so much in this way; we think just of a good man. The good man sacrifices his own interests for others. But in the East they contrast the merely good man with the wise man, who is able to benefit himself as well as others. And the view of Dr. Kano is that you cannot in fact do much good to other people, unless you have cultivated yourself. We tend to think: 'Oh, no, no. Do some good to others. Never mind about yourself'.

In such cases where it is a question of what to think and what to do, Dr. Kano recommended us to study for ourselves. Again and again he says in these writings: 'Study for yourself, do research yourself, find these things out for yourself'. He also said: 'Don't read many books. Read a few really good books and know them minutely, in detail'. One of the subjects he recommended was the study of history. History tells us that many people have thought that they wanted to do good, but that they have failed to think whether they themselves were going to be able to do good.

One of the examples from history was the Roman Emperor who came to the supreme position when he was only 18. He was an artist and a musician, and he wanted to replace the bloodstained triumphs of victorious generals by Triumphs of Art, where the crowns would be given to artists and musicians and dancers. He wanted to make Rome cultured and civilized. He passed a law under which any slave who was ill-treated could appeal to the magistrate, show the mark and ask for the magistrate's protection. The magistrate must then order a compulsory sale of the slave to a good master.

So by that one act the young Emperor took away the fear of torture from the lives of something like a million people—there were probably that number of slaves in the Empire at that time. That was doing good, wasn't it? And yet, in ten years' time he was personally taking part in the tortures himself, because he had not cultivated his own mind, and he became totally sadistic and degraded.

Dr. Kano made a big point of this: benefit others and benefit the self at the same time. He doesn't specify in detail (at least in the parts I have read) what that benefit is, but he says: 'Find it in yourself, cultivate it in yourself. Intelligence should be cultivated in yourself, and the Judo training is really a means of cultivating courage, will and intelligence through these forms of attack and defence'.

He adds that the same things can be learnt in other forms and gives the example of the big department stores in Japan. They were all originally—about 100 years ago—just haberdashery shops; they simply sold cloth. When the Westernization of Japan began, they became these huge department stores like the Selfridge's. But they had all begun in a small way, selling cloth. Dr. Kano explains that it would be a mistake to think that their business success is necessarily tied up with selling that. It was true that they had learnt how to buy and sell by trading in cloth, but then they had extended that knowledge and skill to everything else.

In the same way, Judo must give us qualities which we can use in our daily life, and we must study how to apply what we learn in Judo to our lives.

Bunbu Ryodo 文武両道

A great second principle emphasized by Dr. Kano is *Bunbu Ryodo*. You will recognize two out of the four Japanese characters here: the second character *bu*, or the first character in Budokai, means 'martial' or 'fighting will' and 'courage'; and the last character *do*, or the second character in Judo, means a Way, as distinct from merely a technical skill.

The whole phrase means 'Culture and Martial Power, Both Ways Together'. Now, *bun* means literature and stands for civilization and culture in general; *bu*, as you know, means fighting spirit. Dr. Kano was using a very old ideal in Japan: culture and power united together. Culture without power will be ineffective, and power without culture will be barbarous. Dr. Kano exemplified the ideal in himself; he invented Judo, and then he was a great figure in Japanese education, headmaster of two important colleges and the author of all these writings which are collected in these three big volumes.

The character *bun*, as he explained it, included culture, refinement, good character, and clarity of vision and intelligence. *Bu* means fighting ability, willpower, concentration and the ability to remain calm in a crisis. He divided this character into two parts; he did this with Europeans, and though it may seem a bit complicated, I will do it too. The part at the bottom-left means to 'check' or 'stop', and the part to the top-right was the old character for a 'spear'. So the whole character means to 'check the spear'.

What it means is that one should learn to use a spear not for the purpose of attacking but in order to 'check the spear' with which one is attacked. This was to be the fundamental basis of the *bu* power which you get through practising Judo or other martial arts. The ideal was intelligence and power, and these two Dr. Kano explains with many examples.

Training for What?

Dr. Kano says that we must not specialize in some training without thinking what the training is for. There is an important Confucian saying: 'The true man is not a tool'. He is not an implement. Suppose we are paid to do something, say, to build a bridge. If we neglect the inner culture, the development of our intelligence and will and sense of beauty in our bridge-building, then we are just an implement that builds bridges. In the same way when we teach Judo, we must not just teach technique: we must develop our own intelligence and capacity for thinking.

Judo is an inspiring system of training for life, because in Judo the impossible happens. In about 1903 my father saw Yukio Tani, who had just come to the West. My father was very impressed with Tani's marvellous victories over wrestlers and boxers. Tani was very famous; he appears, for instance, in Bernard Shaw's 1905 play *Major Barbara*, where one character describes how he defeats the local fighters of the East End in London. When my father finally found out that I was doing Judo under Tani, he asked, 'What is he teaching you?' I showed him one or two of the techniques like *kouchi-gari*. My father said, 'Oh no, that's not the real stuff!'

'What do you mean?' I asked.

'I saw him beat a huge man', he replied. 'And he is a small man himself, isn't he? He must have touched some nerve centre to paralyze the huge man; he could never have thrown that big man otherwise. I expect he doesn't teach you the real secrets yet'. My father could not believe that by speed, balance, technique and timing a big man could be thrown by a small man. The impossible happened.

In Judo one of the beauties was that any means could be used—absolutely any—provided that they were not dangerous for the opponent. There weren't all these rules that we have now. And that meant there was a great scope for surprise and the exercise of intelligence. Surprise was very important, but as the rules are increased in number and the possibilities become fewer, it is more and more difficult to surprise anyone. We know everything that can happen: it is like a game of tennis, in which you know everything that can happen. You may not be able to do it, of course. But in Judo, you can practise for 20 years with the best Judo men and still suddenly come across something quite new to you.

The Wide Range and the Short Range

Technique develops, and in a very wide field of possibilities technique can develop almost endlessly. Even in a narrow field, it is wrong to think that the best technique has necessarily been found after a couple of hundred years' experience. We should not become slaves to fixed ideas and analysis of technique.

I learnt the piano as a kid under a teacher of the old school, who was a pupil of the great teacher Oskar Beringer. He taught me to play scales with a matchbox balanced on the back of the hand. I learnt to keep the back of the hand level even when the thumb passes underneath the fingers. I made quite good progress and became able to do it.

And then my father sent me to a very famous teacher, and one of the first things he said to me was, 'Why do you keep your hands so flat?'

'I can balance a matchbox on the back of my hand', I said proudly. I thought he would challenge me to do it, but he said simply, 'What for?'

I didn't know any bad words when I was eight years old, but I thought to myself, 'Oh gosh!' Then he said: 'Throw your hand up when you pass the thumb underneath. Make the wrist soft and throw the hand up. Then it's easier'.

Well, that gave me a lifelong suspicion of fixed rules of technique. But when I had finished laughing at this 20-year-old tradition, I realized that they made good pianists in early days. It may not have been necessary, but they made good pianists. Some of them could play faster than our best people today. It may have been oppressive and unnecessarily difficult, but it did get results too. One thinks that one can analyze technique and get it out straight, once for all; one thinks that one now knows the best way. But it doesn't necessarily follow.

Another point which Dr. Kano discusses is the question of short term and long term. He writes that we must retain clearly our final objective, but also that we must be able to concentrate on what is immediately before us.

There is a wide range, and there is also a short range, and we must be able to direct attention accordingly. We can see this in golf. When they first play golf, beginners make the stroke, but before they have actually hit the ball, they are looking up to see where it has gone. As a result, they miss it altogether. To play a golf shot you first have to get a wide span of attention: the direction, how far to hit the ball, where it will pitch, what effect the slopes will have, and so on. You get a feeling in your body of how the stroke is to be. When you actually hit the ball, you don't think of any of these consequences; you just hit the ball with that feeling in your body.

Look at the photos of the great tournament professionals, and you will see that most of them are still looking down at where the ball was, long after it has been despatched. They do not look up, even after hitting the ball. But beginners are looking up even before they have hit it. The beginners make up their mind not to look up, but still they do so. They cannot control the impulse to look up. In this way, the extra unnecessary thought interferes with the stroke, and many golfers spend their whole lives looking up before they hit the ball. They never succeed in controlling the impulse, because they have no mental control. They resolve to keep their head down, but up it comes.

Judo in Real Life

Mental control is a very important part of Judo training. We need courage. We haven't had a war here—a major war—for a long time, but people who have been through some of the worst of war say that a Judo contest can sometimes be more frightening than actual danger. To that extent our contests are a very good training. It's not a question of being frightened but still going through. That's something inferior. If the training is pursued, there is an inner calmness. When we face something very extreme— perhaps death, perhaps something even more unpleasant— then we shall know whether our Judo training has been going really deep.

Perhaps you may suffer a medical catastrophe, while you are still young. The doctor looks at all the results of the tests and examinations, and says, 'Oh'. And you will ask, 'How long will it be before I get better?'

'Some of these cases make progress', he replies.

'What about mine?'

'Well, it's only afterwards really that we can tell: that was a good one, that was a bad one', the doctor says.

You don't really get more out of him, but if you know a consultant personally, perhaps you go to him and say: 'What are the chances in these cases? I want to know'.

'One in five will survive', he says.

Perhaps that's not so easy to meet. But if we have practised Judo in the full sense, then it will slowly come to help us. And maybe when on another occasion we come back home and find our house has been gutted by fire, it may turn out that we are not nearly so upset as might be expected.

When Dr. Kano was in Italy, he was travelling in a coach through the mountains, and one of the members of the Japanese embassy was with him. The coach went off the road and stopped halfway over the edge of a cliff, and there was a hysterical panic among some of the passengers. But that man from the embassy told us: 'Dr. Kano was quite calm. He knew it might go over any second, but he sat there quietly. That helped to restore quiet among the passengers, and they came off quietly'.

What Judo Teaches Us

We have to become able to meet disadvantages. In most sports, if there is some injury, people say, 'Oh, you can't expect me to go on; I've got a bad elbow' or whatever it is. But in Judo we are trained to go on even with injuries. We know that the body is only 30 percent effective, perhaps only 20 percent effective. But we are not demoralized, and we can use the remaining 30 percent or 20 percent, whereas many people, if they are injured or feel a little sick, cannot do anything at all. They are completely knocked out.

The ability to keep up morale in the face of disadvantages can be a great help for our lives. There is a saying in Japan, 'Every man has seven faults'. Well, to know that we have faults but to go on in spite of those faults, to find ways of lessening them and avoid having those faults completely destroy our lives—Judo would help us with that, if we think back to the times when we have been injured. Not demoralized. Injured but not demoralized.

We have to become resourceful and we have to become objective. An expert on the ground whom I saw and knew at the Kodokan was a vicious man. He used to put the locks on and just put them on a little bit more to hurt. He did not do any damage, he never caused any injury at all, but he would just hurt. He was an expert on locks on the ground, and in those days the rules were wider, so there were more locks.

Well, I practised with him. I could throw him some times, but on the ground he was much better. I experienced this and saw him hurting other people. No one liked to practise with him, and I was among them. But then I realized: 'No, I'm wrong. He's a most unpleasant man, and it's not very nice to have these little pains, but you can learn a lot'. I did practise with him regularly, and as a matter of fact after a time he stopped doing it.

Another thing which Judo can teach us is: 'Hold tightly, let go lightly'. Suppose I am holding this stick tightly. You would have to be quite strong to make me let go in the ordinary way. But if someone comes along who knows, he can just press the end of the stick in exactly the right direction. I may be holding like mad, but sooner or later the pain at the root of the thumb is going to be too bad. I am forced down and out of balance trying to hold on, but in the end I have to let go. And my balance has been destroyed, and my hand hurts.

In general, if we are holding an opponent and he moves in the right way and gets out, to continue trying to hold on and on, one's own position is ruined. In these cases we should hold tightly, but when we can see that it's going, let go abruptly and even push it away.

Then we retain the balance, and we can turn and move freely in a good position to meet whatever may happen next. For this can happen in life. We must apply this in life. We try something very hard, put all we have into it. Then it begins to go, to leave us. We think: 'No, no. I'll hold on. Don't go, don't go'. But it goes, and we are left regretting; our balance, so to speak, has been destroyed. Instead of that, Judo can teach us to let go, even cheerfully to push it away, 'Go, then'. Judo can teach us how to do that.

Being Good on the Mat Isn't Enough

In these writings Dr. Kano often says, 'Find these applications of Judo to your daily life, and don't just practise Judo on the mat'.

When we fall in Judo, the first thing we learn is to fall with the whole body. If one tries, as the beginner does, to keep off the ground, then the whole shock comes on to one unfortunate wrist or elbow, which gets badly hurt. The right technique is not to try to keep off the ground but to take the fall with all of us.

In the same way, when we have a failure in life, try to use our Judo experience and take that failure. But people tend to say, 'Oh, wasn't I unlucky?' or 'It was their fault; they let me down' or more often 'Well, I wasn't feeling very well then, you know'. Dr. Tartakower, who was a great chess master but had been in his youth a Hungarian cavalry officer and a famous duelist, once remarked, 'I've never beaten a man, either at chess or in a duel, who was wholly well'.

We have to develop faith, faith in ourselves. Judo can give us faith. We are able to have faith, even when we are trying something where we seem to have no chance at all. In the Kodokan in the old days they used to be ranged in groups round the wall; all the 4th dans stood together, and all the 5th dans and so on. The grades tended to practise mostly in their own groups, and when you moved up a grade, you come into a new group. Perhaps you would go on first with some hard-bitten trap-scarred veteran of that group. (He would never move up any more, but in his group he would be very formidable. In a way these chaps were like rungs of a ladder; they had a fixed position, and you had to move up past them, if you could.)

Now the first time you go on with a man like that, it isn't that you can't throw him: you can't shift him. And then you think, 'Oh for goodness' sake, you know I've been doing Judo for seven years, and I can't shift him. He is like the Rock of Gibraltar'. But you have faith in yourself, so you practise with him every day. And then one afternoon, you find that he has got a weakness. Yes, he has got a weakness. And then you find you can exploit that weakness, and after three months, yes you can sometimes throw him. And after six months you can throw him a lot, and after nine months, it's not worth practising with him. That gives you faith—faith in yourself.

When you have got a little bit of experience like that, then it has to be applied, as Dr. Kano said, to our own lives:

'Oh, I'm no good at calculations, mathematics. Can't add up or do anything. Now I am put into an office and I've got to add columns and columns of six-figure numbers. And now I'm liable to think that I just can't do that, no I can't'.

'But I have to do it, so I do it slowly with many mistakes, and I have to check it and check it again and get somebody else to check it as well. I may go on and on like that, always frightened by it, always making a mess of it, always trying to get out of it'.

But a true Judo man doesn't do that. He faces it, just as he faced that veteran whom he couldn't throw. He goes out and buys a little book on rapid calculations, and he practises for 20 minutes every morning and evening. In three or four weeks he becomes a master of rapid calculation. The very thing he was so frightened of he masters completely. In these ways Judo can help our lives, not just be something which we are good at on the mat.

The Spirit of Budo

The Will to Make It Happen

Now let me talk about an example which doesn't apply to anyone else here. Suppose I am 60 and I want to learn a new and difficult language. People would tell me: 'That's absolutely out, absolutely out! At your age, you know, the brain cells are dying at the rate of 100,000 a day'. I look it up, and it's true. I feel like clutching my head and crying, 'Aaargh!' That's what they want me to do. But if I have faith, I think that I can do it with fewer brain cells and then find that in fact I can.

As a matter of fact, if I look a bit deeper I find that I've got 10,000,000,000 brain cells, so at that rate they'll last me 274 years. If I had been scared off, I should have been scared by nothing.

In this sort of way, the experiences which we have at Judo are meant to be a training for later experiences in life. If we just practise and teach Judo, as something separate from life, then it is really probably not worth spending very much time in it. It is interesting, but not all that interesting. But if we can combine it—and perhaps in our teaching show others how to combine it—with living experience, that is something important and valuable.

The Impossible Can Happen

One of the artists of the early part of this century was Eric Gill, and he remarked that in Britain we tend to think of art as something where you have to get out your easel, you get out your oils and you paint a lovely picture. Then you go and do something else.

'So, art must be brought into our everyday lives', said Gill. For instance, he designed new typefaces, so that art would be brought into what we are reading. His design, called Gill Sans, is very famous, and when we read something printed in it, we receive a vague impression of something beautiful. Perhaps we don't know why that book or whatever it is gives an attractive impression, but it does.

Judo can be brought into the smallest things in our daily lives. People often hold a pen near the very tip, so that they have to keep shifting their hand on the paper every word or so. And they hold it very tightly—often you can see the white round the tips of the fingers. But a pen has length and should be held well up its length, balanced on the fingers even if the thumb is taken away for a moment. Then when you write, you don't have to keep shifting the hand. An expert high-speed shorthand writer holds it like that.

The Judo principle of maximum efficiency can teach us many things about our most ordinary activities. Dr. Kano insisted that what you learn in your interesting Judo practice must affect your daily life.

For example, when we are teaching a beginner on the ground, sometimes we pass our left hand from behind under his chin and hold his right *eri*, high up by the side of his neck. Then we come forward and show our face to him on his right side. He sees us, and of course he wants to get at us to fight us. So he turns to the right. And as he turns so strongly to the right, he strangles himself. It sometimes takes him quite a little time to realize that he should turn away, and that will release the pressure. He should whirl away, and then he is free to come back at us.

Something very similar often happens in life. We are trying to get something, and we try very directly. But somehow, we seem to be killing ourselves doing it. When we apply our Judo experience, we realize we must turn away—turn away abruptly and completely. Then we are free to come back. Often we find that we only succeed in getting things when we are free to turn completely away. Not so easy. But Dr. Kano says that it is in just these things that the value and interest of Judo training lie.

Again, Judo can show us how to look at limitations. Limitations, we are told, must be accepted. They tell us that we have all got limitations, and we must accept them. Judo shows us—as many other things in life can show us too if we look—that the limitations at the beginning can be changed. Even what the expert may point out to you as 'your limitations' can be changed.

Edith Evans, one of our greatest actresses, was rejected by the teachers at an important drama school at her first hearing. In her reminiscences she says: 'Yes, they gave me a hearing. And then they told me, "Well, no"'. But she became a genius at acting. If she had accepted that 'limitation' which they thought she had, it would have been a great loss.

I knew very well the Japanese *shogi* (chess) champion Yasuharu Oyama. Chess is a much more popular game in Japan than it is here, and the chess champion is as big a national figure as a football star here.

When Oyama was a small boy, he got the idea that he wanted to play and went to a famous *dojo* training hall in Osaka. They gave him a few test games. The head teacher, a man of enormous experience who trained champions, told him: 'My boy, you haven't got the talent for it. To take you on as an apprentice wouldn't be honest, and it wouldn't be fair to you. You haven't got the basic gift for this—go and try something else'.

Well, Oyama, the little boy, wept and finally the teacher said: 'Look, I'm not taking you on as a pupil, because that would not be fair to you. If you like, after school you can come here and you can help clean up, as a servant. You can watch the games and you can play occasionally, but I'm not taking you on as a student. It would be wrong and would just give you false hopes'.

Oyama became champion at least ten times, and he dominated Japanese chess for 25 years. He won 100 major competitions in those 25 years. If he had accepted that decision about his limitations, he would have failed.

Judo can teach us this: things which are impossible for us can happen. Things one would think absolutely impossible can come about, if intelligence and will are applied.

Emptying the Mind

One of Dr. Kano's main themes is that we should study. 'Far more important than studying by books', he says, 'is actually to study for oneself'. Books ought to have a government health warning on them; they are addictive and they can seriously damage your health. Study and find out for yourselves, not secondhand. He said that the *kata* or pattern should be studied in its traditional forms, but he added that new *kata* must be developed.

People tend to think, 'Tell us what to do, because we don't know'. No, study and find things out for yourselves. There is inspiration if we can control the mind. Traditionally, after the Judo practice they used to practise controlling the mind. They practised sitting quite still for five or ten minutes, pouring with sweat or maybe blood, but not moving.

'Really? What's the use of that?' people ask. A great use. From the ability to empty the mind inspiration comes. First intense study, and then emptying of the mind, which takes a lot of control.

Linus Pauling, a double Nobel Prize winner with a string of important discoveries to his credit (and in his old age he has just now discovered a new form of chemical bond), says this about his method:

'For dealing with problems that initially defeat me, I deliberately make use of my subconscious mind. I think about the problem when going to bed, and in bed, for a week or two. Then I deliberately dismiss it from my mind and forget it. Then weeks or months later, as with the structure of alphakeratin (which was one of his discoveries) the answer suddenly pops into my mind complete'.

He studies hard and then deliberately forgets it; that takes great control. Something one has concentrated on to just dismiss it from the mind.

We can have inspiration in Judo; it can come suddenly. But to cultivate it systematically, the mind has to be controlled and that practice in silent sitting is one of the ways of learning to control the mind.

Notes

1. Kaiten Nukariya (1876-1934), a noted Buddhist philosopher and a Zen priest. In 1924, he became president of Komazawa University.
2. Dr. Jigoro Kano was born in 1860 and graduated from Tokyo Imperial University in 1881, where he majored in literature and political science. In the following year he founded the Kodokan for the study and instruction of Judo. In later years he became principal of Gakushuin and Tokyo Higher Normal School. In 1889 he visited Europe to study educational institutions there as a member of the Imperial Household Department. He became the first Japanese member of the International Olympic Committee in 1909. He died in 1938 on his return voyage from Cairo where he attended an IOC meeting.
3. Saigo Takamori (1827-1877), a leader in the overthrow of the Tokugawa shogunate and the creation of the Meiji government. His statue stands in Ueno Park in Tokyo, showing him as a man of the common people, dressed in a casual kimono with his favorite dog at his side.
4. Junjiro Takakusu (1866-1945), a philosopher of Buddhism, professor of the University of Tokyo and author of numerous books on Buddhism.
5. *Itto-ryu*, a leading school of swordsmanship in the Edo period. It was named after the founder, Ito Ittosai Kagehisa.
6. Hojo Tokimune (1251-1284). When faced with the threat of Mongolian invaders, he fortified northwestern Kyushu and successfully repelled them in 1274 and 1281.
7. *Shonan katto-roku*, an anecdote about Buddhism and feudal warriors, included in a book edited by Fukuzan Imai (1924), a Buddhist priest in Kyushu.

8. Katsu Kaishu (1823-1899), a statesman who was active in the transition from the Tokugawa shogunate to the Meiji government. In boyhood, he was trained in swordsmanship.
9. Yamaoka Tesshu (1836-1888), a swordsman and retainer of the Tokugawa shogunate. In later years he served as an aide to the Meiji Emperor.
10. Oda Nobunaga (1534-1582), the principal figure who reunified Japan in the 16th century when it was riven by civil war.
11. Hachiko, known as 'Chuken Hachiko', or 'Hachiko, the faithful dog'. For 10 long years in the early Showa era, Hachiko paid daily visits to the Shibuya Station in Tokyo to meet his master, not aware that he had already passed away. The dog's unflagging devotion to his master impressed many Japanese. In the mid-1930s, a bronze statue of Hachiko was erected on the west side of the station; it is still a popular landmark in Tokyo. The real Hachiko was stuffed and is now on display at the National Science Museum, Tokyo.
12. Daidoji Yuzan (1639-1730), a military strategist born in Kyoto. In *Budo shoshin-shu* he provides brilliant practical insights into the essence of Budo.
13. *Shinno shintoryu,* an influential school of Kendo founded in the late 15th century.

Glossary

dan, grade. Those ranking first through fifth dan wear black belts. For sixth through eighth dan the belt has red-and-white stripes. Ninth dan and above wear a red belt.

harai-goshi, hip sweep

ippon. The referee announces 'ippon' when a contestant throws his opponent largely on his back, when a contestant holds his opponent for 30 seconds, or when a contestant gives up by tapping two or three times with his hand or foot.

jujutsu, an old form of traditional Japanese martial arts, which unlike contemporary Judo involved hitting, kicking, stabbing and slashing.

kouchi-gari, small inner reap

osoto-gari, large outer reap

randori, free practice

tsurikomi, lifting and pulling

waza-ari. The referee announces 'waza-ari' when a contestant throws his opponent but when the technique is not sufficient to qualify the attacker for *ippon*.

Other books by Trevor Leggett

Championship Judo (with Kisaburo Watanabe)
Kata Judo (with Dr Jigoro Kano)
Samurai Zen (The Warrior Koans)
Zen and The Ways
Three Ages of Zen
A First Zen Reader
A Second Zen Reader (The Tiger's Cave)
Japanese Chess (Shogi: Japan's Game of Strategy)
Encounters in Yoga and Zen
Lotus Lake, Dragon Pool
Jewels from the Indra Net
Fingers and Moons
The Old Zen Master
The Chapter of the Self
Realisation of the Supreme Self
The Complete Commentary by Śaṅkara on the Yoga Sūtra-s
The Dragon Mask

THE SPIRIT OF BUDO

www.ingramcontent.com/pod-product-compliance
Lightning Source LLC
Chambersburg PA
CBHW071528080526
44588CB00011B/1597